PROMISCUOUS EATING

PROMISCUOUS EATING

*Understanding and Ending
Our Self-Destructive Relationship
with Food*

Andrew Siegel, M.D.

March 2011

To Kathy — all the best.
Thank you for your help (in advance) —
hopefully there will be plenty of
book buying going on at the front
of the office!   Andy

Published by ROGUE WAVE PRESS

Copyright © 2011 by Andrew L. Siegel, M.D.

The Library of Congress Cataloging-in-Publication has been applied for.

Printed in the United States of America
First printing 2011

ISBN: 978-0-9830617-0-0

To order additional copies of this book:

www.promiscuouseating.com

DISCLAIMER: This publication contains the opinions, ideas, and biases of the author. There is no intent that any of the information provided should be construed as medical advice or professional medical services. Before adopting recommendations made in the book, it is imperative that you consult with your own health care provider. The author and publisher disclaim any and all responsibility for any liability or loss incurred as a consequence of the use of any of the information provided.

*This book is dedicated to my children—
Jeffrey, Alexa, and Isabelle. Jeff is a child of
my 20's, Lex of my 30's, and Belle of my
40's. With age clearly has come a better
and keener appreciation of these unique,
distinctive and special creatures who never
cease to astonish me.*

Contents

Acknowledgments   ix

Preface   xi

Introduction   xix

Chapter 1   THE PROBLEM: *Uber*-Eating in
the United States of *Obesity*   1

Chapter 2   THE SKINNY ON WHY WE EAT   9

Chapter 3   WHAT FOODS TO BE WARY OF:
Caveat Emptor (Buyer Beware)   33

Chapter 4   PSYCHOLOGICAL PERSPECTIVES:
The Mind Vis-à-Vis Eating—
Battling Raw Emotions with Food   61

Chapter 5   SOLUTIONS: Chew Over These Ideas   81

Appendix 1   RAW FACTS AND TRUTHS   113

Appendix 2   100 VALUABLE NUGGETS AND TIDBITS   123

Recommended Resources   129

Acknowledgments

Thank you first and foremost to Les, my faithful partner, steadfast helpmate, collaborator, confidante, editor and best friend. She is a rather "low maintenance" wife, and has always been an unwavering advocate and unconditional supporter. She has never begrudged me the substantial amounts of personal time I have spent pursuing my desires (so my envious friends tell me!). Her years of experience in the publishing field as an editor at Prentice Hall and a publishing executive at Random House prior to becoming a mom and the CEO of our household have proven invaluable to me in terms of converting my sometimes tangential rambling into coherent prose and medical mumbo-jumbo into readable English. She has been a source of clarity, solace and sustenance and a loving and stalwart fixture in my existence in a world too often marked by randomness, chaos, and lunacy.

Thank you to all of you who graciously and generously allowed me a brief and perhaps annoying intrusion into your lives with a barrage of questions about your eating habits and the particulars of what triggers non-hunger-driven eating. By revealing very personal and intimate details and secrets, you have provided me with a bounty of real life and practical information that supplied much of the material for this book. For this, my appreciation is boundless. Fictional names have been tagged to your quotes to protect your privacy. Some quotes are verbatim while others have been edited and condensed in an effort to maintain fluidity while keeping the content and sentiment intact.

Finally, thank you to *you*, the reader, for taking the time from your lives to spend with my words. My goal is that these pages may serve to contribute to your health, wellness and mindfulness and, ultimately, to an improved relationship with food that will help you achieve or maintain the weight and well being that you desire.

Preface

Among my patients to whom I provide medical care, I have witnessed a clear correlation between a healthy lifestyle and a healthy existence. I have recognized the importance of nutritious, wholesome and natural foods in terms of health maintenance and disease prevention, and likewise, the very negative impact of poor eating on our health and wellness.

For as long as I can remember, I have been interested in maximizing my *own* health and well being through an intelligent lifestyle including exercise, prudent food choices, and the avoidance of tobacco. I attempt to work out daily and am usually very careful about the food that I consume. I make a concerted effort to eat ample amounts of whole grain products, fruits, vegetables and legumes, to eat animal products in moderation, and to avoid fast and processed foods. That being said, I confess to having more moments than I care to admit when I have found myself consuming unnecessary, unhealthy, inappropriate, unwarranted calories and junk. This is in spite of my being a rather disciplined, tightly controlled, type A personality.

It is only recently that rather than just chastise myself for these indiscretions, I began to think about why I behave in this manner. I attempted to deconstruct the reasons behind my occasional meanders of mindless consumption of manufactured muck. I endeavored to apply more mindfulness to both the rationale and motivations underpinning my momentary lapses as well as to the specifics of my food choices.

At times I find myself staring inside the refrigerator or pantry, mindlessly foraging for something to eat, even though I am not hungry and may even have just eaten. I wonder to myself, what am I doing here? It seems that I am searching for something more profound than

*food, but I'm not sure what that is. At these times, I am often aware
that my consciousness is altered, as I am in a somewhat muddled and
stuporous state of mind, gazing forward without really seeing. If I can
muster up the gumption to shake myself out of that state and sharpen
my self-awareness and mindfulness, I can exit the scene without consuming needless and unwanted calories that will be regretted later.
There always exists a moment when I can give in or resist and retreat.*

I have always been more physical than metaphysical, more
swayed by the tangible than the intangible, more of a realist and a
pragmatist than a dreamer. Proceeding against my natural grain, I re-
solved to "expand my horizons" through self-education as well as
yoga and meditation classes, which is where I was really first exposed to the concept of *mindfulness*. I came to understand that pro-
ficiency in the art of being mindful does not come naturally and
demands cultivation.

My interest in refining my own mindfulness converged with a
curiosity and passion for the disciplines of food and nutrition, important topics given short shrift in medical school. I came to appreciate that simply by carefully reading food labels, significant insight
can be obtained regarding the component ingredients and their nutritional values or lack thereof. I realized that what we eat could,
on a certain level, be thought of in similar terms as *medication*, demanding wise and judicious usage. I recognized that we are on an
absolute need-to-know basis about precisely what it is that we are
consuming. I made it my business to learn everything I could about
the science of food and nutrition, particularly about processed foods
with their unhealthy triad of components—*enriched wheat flour,
partially hydrogenated vegetable oil,* and *high fructose corn syrup*—
ubiquitous in our diets, having addictive properties, and potentially
as malignant as tobacco.

I started thinking more about my own *food choices* and also
about my own *eating behavior*. I gave serious consideration as to
why I eat for reasons other than being genuinely hungry. I became
more aware of my state of mind when eating and concluded that my
own consumption was, at times, emotionally driven as opposed to
being hunger driven, and that this eating-for-the-wrong-reason resulted in the needless consumption of excessive calories. It occurred
to me that if two thirds of the American population is overweight or
obese, then many of us are likely impelled to eat on the basis of this

mindless, emotionally-driven behavior, aside from the poor food choices that many of us make.

I am fortunate to be in respectable physical shape and not overweight, although I do work hard at my fitness. I consume plenty of calories—although generally through very healthy foods—but I compensate by being an avid exerciser who rarely misses a day. I do feel that when I eat I do not achieve satiety as many others do, and after eating a seemingly adequate volume of food, I am just not all that full, and usually stop because I am conscious of how much I have consumed and at a certain point must just say "enough." Like many others, I am prone to eating when I am not hungry and this is clearly dysfunctional and unhealthy. Introspection applied to my own eating patterns brought forth some interesting insights.

Why do I eat when I am not hungry? Like so many of us, I experience a significant amount of *stress* at work. I see a lot of patients, there is a great deal of multi-tasking and juggling involved, difficult decisions, etc., and I am left not only physically and emotionally depleted but also rather tense. Under these circumstances, food becomes a very soothing antidote, and I sometimes fall prey to its medicinal effects. Interestingly, I have found exercise to be an alternative and equally effective means of dealing with the pressures and anxieties of life, doing wonders for ameliorating the stress in a more appropriate and healthy fashion than mindless eating.

As I was driving to work one day thinking about emotional and mindless eating, I turned on the radio and I heard the Ramones belting out the lyrics: "I Wanna Be Sedated." I had an epiphany-like revelation that the essence of what many of us seek when we eat not out of genuine hunger—but for emotional reasons—is a form of sedation from the many stresses, hassles, worries, tensions, difficulties and burdens of our daily existence.

What else drives my mindless and unnecessary eating? For me, *alcohol* does the trick but good. On an evening when I have a glass or two of wine or beer with dinner (I rarely drink any other liquor), I find myself foraging for food shortly after dinner. What is it about alcohol that fosters this pattern of mindless and dysfunctional eating? I believe it is simply that alcohol releases inhibitions that cause my eating "guard" to drop down low enough to engender this behavior; my discipline has simply been subverted by alcohol. More on this later.

For me, another one of the key triggers of mindless eating is *fatigue*. Physically, mentally and emotionally weary from a long day of work, sometimes too tired to read or really be attentive to anything demanding, I find myself in an altered state of mind. I might vegetate in front of the television, mindlessly consuming something, not particularly enjoying the eating experience but nonetheless continuing the behavior in relentless fashion, until the job is complete. I gaze at the empty bowl, questioning why I consumed without being driven by hunger and without much pleasure or any redemptive value to the eating. When I apply some thought to the situation, I realize that mindless watching of television is little different from mindless eating. I conclude that somehow my fatigue overrides my normal reasonably tight control over my behaviors and that what I really need is not food to stimulate my taste buds nor the visual and auditory stimulation of television...I simply require a good night's rest. So, I am at times substituting mindless eating and mindless television consumption for rest and sleep.

Last evening, I had a bout of mindless eating. I was tired and spent, just back to work for the first day after a vacation. The office was very busy and I had expended a great deal of emotional energy being a careful listener and making an effort to be as sympathetic and empathetic to my patients as possible. Upon arriving home, I exercised, showered, and had a healthy dinner with my family—wild salmon over whole wheat pasta, a salad, and a nice glass of Sauvignon Blanc to drink. After dinner, I worked on my computer for an hour or so, did The New York Times crossword, and decided to watch some television. In the family room, I turned on the winter Olympics and grabbed a healthy snack—an apple—'no harm done there.' I observed my wife eating almonds and they just looked so enticing that I acted upon my urge and obtained one of those 100 calorie packs of dry roasted almonds—'okay, still not so bad—plenty of healthy fats and not so many calories.' Then I had a hankering for something else, so I went foraging in the pantry and discovered a large container of honey wheat braided pretzel twists—'yum—so I counted out seven on a paper plate, which is one serving, 110 calories.' After downing these, I noticed my daughter eating a few peanut M & M's. She left the box on the coffee table in front of me, and I stared at that tempting yellow box as I watched some crazy, high-adrenaline Olympic event that looked like high diving, except on skis and without a pool. I thought to myself, 'well, I'll just have one.' And one I did, and then a few more, and then a few more—not a terrible amount, but still, totally gratuitous and unnecessary. It almost seemed that it wasn't me eating, but my alter ego eating. I constructed a mental image of a plate with the contents of my snacking—an apple, a serving of almonds, seven pretzels, and a handful of M & M's—and felt a bit disgusted. I surfed through some channels and proceeded to doze off on the couch.

The following morning, after a great night's rest, I was able to truly think about my previous evening's "misconduct." I hadn't really given it a great deal of thought the evening before, aside from picturing the contents of my "binge" on an imaginary plate, a bizarre habit I have developed when I overdo it with eating. There is nothing like a refreshed and clear head to foster some serious introspection, and my mental status the evening before was anything but perky and lucid. The forces that seemed to impel my eating were a combination of exhaustion, wine, the reflex turn-on-the-television-go-to-the-pantry-nocturnal noshing habit that I have a tendency for, as well as the temptation from watching my wife munch away on crunchy almonds and the opportunity from the box of M & M's sitting within grasp. Usually disciplined, strong willed and nutritionally conscientious, I simply had a bit of a stumble to the realm of mindless eating. I really wasn't hungry and didn't take much pleasure in the act. It would seem that I can be a fallible, imperfect and weak-willed human as, of course, we all are at times. I can easily rationalize the apple and the almonds as 200 calories worth of a healthy snack. The pretzels and M & M's were an unnecessary additional few hundred calories. I should have just gone upstairs and gone to sleep! Was a few hundred extra calories of indulgence going to do me in? Perhaps, if I did so on a regular basis, but I rarely overdo it like that. If I think long-term-big-picture perspective, I merely had a little deviation off the pathway on the journey towards good health and fitness, and I vowed to make a concerted effort to "behave better" in the future as well as to stay active and continue my exercise regimen.

Another trigger of mindless eating for me is being in a bad mood:

About two months after having experienced the epiphany from hearing "I Wanna Be Sedated," I was driving in my car on a Sunday morning when I heard the Ramones singing "I Don't Care." I don't know what it is about the Ramones' lyrics that get my mind going, but that set me into thinking about my eating behavior the evening before. That Saturday afternoon, I had played tennis for the first time in a month, given that I had recently had a ventral hernia repair. After tennis, I sat with my buddies chatting and found myself in a nasty mood—really kind of rare for me. My shoulder, which might need to be operated on, was hurting, my abdominal incision was smarting, and I was unhappy with my performance on the court. To boot, I received an annoying and disturbing telephone call, which further set me off. When I arrived home in an ill-tempered mood, I sat down with my wife to a healthy chili dinner (ground turkey substituted for beef). I proceeded to eat way too many pieces of sourdough bread and returned to the chili pot FOUR times for generous refills that I ladled into my bowl!

I simply had way too much to eat and I was totally aware of that fact, but I was in such a malignant mood that I just didn't care. It seemed that my mood clouded my eating judgment and permitted a temporary lapse of eating sanity, and the eating served as comfort and consolation for my ill humor. So, my usual mindfulness was undermined by the altered state induced by my cantankerous mood.

My introspection regarding my own bouts of emotional and mindless eating stimulated me to ask others about their eating behaviors. I arbitrarily planned on interviewing about 100 or so people, but after about 75, the answers started becoming repetitive and redundant. I asked most everybody I came in contact with—young, old, male, female, thin, overweight—if they would answer a few questions regarding their eating habits. I queried family members, friends, office employees, colleagues, hospital and surgical center employees, pharmaceutical and device representatives, etc. This was by no means a rigorous scientific study, but was more of an informal survey. Nonetheless, I feel that I garnered very valuable information. Only a very small percentage of people I solicited were not interested in participating. The key questions were the following:

- *Under what circumstances do you eat when not genuinely hungry?*
- *What do you eat under these circumstances?*
- *If eating for emotional reasons, does the eating provide a sense of relief?*
- *Do you feel guilt or remorse after, and if so, what do you do about it?*

Most people readily opened up to me to reveal their particular triggers to eating when not hungry. The triggers for eating when not physically hungry are most often certain emotional states of mind, but also eating driven by circumstances that I label as follows: *recreational; opportunistic; temptation; accessory; reward; social; deprivation; boredom; fatigue; drug-induced; habit; holiday/tradition; seasonal; hormonal.* On rare occasions, eating occurs in the absence of hunger in order to purposely avoid skipping a meal or to forcibly increase caloric and protein intake for an underweight person or an athlete trying to bulk up muscles.

During the interview process, it became apparent to me that just the very act of opening up, bringing these issues to the forefront and discussing them, was *therapeutic* and *cathartic* for many, even after a relatively brief dialogue. It would seem that many of us bring our emotions "to the table" with respect to eating. In response to most of the negative emotions that we experience over the course of our day-to-day activities, many of us consume foods that we do not want to eat, in excessive quantities. That being said, a fair number of us experience an emotionally driven loss of appetite.

I found that mindless/emotional eating transcends age, race, gender, body shape or weight. Many of the stories were fascinating and compelling. So I organized and analyzed my notes and voilà— practical and real life information about what drives our eating behavior. Many of us eat mindlessly because of the emotional baggage that we bear on any particular day, and this behavior clearly engenders weight gain and possibly obesity. It follows that if this is the case, then the solution to the problem of mindless/emotional eating is the cultivation of a mindful eating strategy, which is much of the basis of the following pages.

Introduction

This is not another diet book. My ambition is to have the reader come to an understanding of his or her own eating behavior in order to change it for the better. For long-term and permanent weight loss to occur, we must comprehend the intricacies of our own unique interrelation with food and modify that relationship—forever more—so that it is a more harmonious one. My intention is to provide strategies to recognize and repair our often uncivil and unfriendly relationship with food that has literally gone awry, in order to enable us to relate to food in a healthy manner. In many cases, food is not the problem, nor is overeating—it is often our thoughts and emotions that are the root cause of this discordant alliance with food. It is not so much what we are consuming, but what emotions are consuming us. Eating is frequently driven by an appetite for the positive feelings derived from the consumption of food and not for an appetite for food itself. It is essential to figure out precisely what emotional needs are being fulfilled by eating and ultimately to learn better ways of dealing with them.

Whether underweight, morbidly obese or anywhere in the gamut in-between, it is never too late to revamp and amend our relationship with food. If we can do so, our diets and eating habits can change considerably, and the health ramifications of these changes can be transformative, if not life saving. Although not easy, it is very much within the realm of possibility. We can remedy our profligate ways. It can be done! Read on.

It is astonishing that two thirds of Americans are either overweight or obese. Weight gain is often brought on by emotional, mindless and *promiscuous* eating patterns based upon this unhealthy relationship with food. Obesity is often a collateral effect of this dysfunctional means of dealing with our emotional "baggage." We literally wear the footprint of stress and other negative emotions on our bodies. Our bodies at any given time largely represent the sum total of all of our food consumption integrated with the sum total of all our physical activity or lack thereof. And for many of us, it is not a pretty picture! This is a very detrimental state of affairs, both for the individual who is carrying the extra pounds and for our nation, on the verge of financial insolvency. A good portion of America's economic woes are predicated upon health care expenses that are as bloated as those whose corpulence—and the health care ramifications of such—is, in a large way, responsible. It has been estimated that about two thirds of the health care expenses of the USA go to pay for preventable, chronic conditions that are directly related to obesity—including diabetes, heart disease, and some cancers. Genetics and bad luck notwithstanding, our lifestyle matters—big time!

Here is a brief story about Dr. Frances Collins, the NIH (National Institutes of Health) chief. Dr. Collins availed himself of new genetic tests that can reveal our genome (hereditary blueprint) and our risk for a number of diseases. It turned out that he had a genetic predisposition for diabetes. So what did he do? He lost 20 pounds by eliminating junk foods, increasing his consumption of fruits and vegetables, and integrating physical activity into his very busy life. Now he feels great and has lessened his risk for diabetes. The bottom line is that "genes load the gun, but lifestyle pulls the trigger" and that the overwhelming majority of us have the capacity to alter our health destiny by modifying our lifestyle in terms of eating and exercise.

Some of us "eat to live," while others "live to eat." Either way, we must all consume food in order to survive. On a daily basis, we make choices regarding the quantity and quality of foods that we ingest, and it is these selections that can ultimately "make or break" us. We can choose to promote our health and well being or, alternatively, we can decide to undermine it. It is abundantly clear that what and how much we decide to place in our mouths can, quite literally, have life or death implications. Unfortunately, many of us make the wrong choices in terms of the foods that we eat—literally *poisoning* our systems with bad foods and/or *flooding* our bodies with excessive amounts of "fuel"—all with devastating consequences. As a physician, I am a direct observer of the havoc wreaked by sub-optimal food and lifestyle choices that result in preventable problems responsible for needless suffering—weight gain, obesity, diabetes, high blood pressure, cardiovascular diseases, cancer, and a myriad of other health issues.

Although we have been given the miraculous gift of life, nonetheless, many of us have been inadequate caretakers of ourselves. Many of us have been remiss in pursuing a nurturing lifestyle, in eating moderately and in consuming robust and wholesome foods that promote vigorous health. When we eat for the wrong reasons—as many of us do—the foods that we ingest under these circumstances are often poor in choice and excessive in volume, which can eventually result in ill health. So, the quality and quantity of what we eat will clearly affect the quality and quantity of our lives.

We must all claim personal responsibility for the stewardship of our own selves. If not us, then whom? As Randy Pausch stated in *The Last Lecture*: "*We cannot change the cards we are dealt, just how we play the hand.*" Since life is short, we should play the hand in as fulfilling, far-reaching and meaningful a way as possible, honoring and respecting ourselves and living the healthiest existence conceivable. We all have within ourselves the ability to cultivate the degree of mindfulness necessary to achieve this.

Many of us lack the knowledge of the salutary benefits of healthy eating and the detrimental effects of unhealthy eating. Many of us are not nutritionally *conscientious* or even nutritionally conscious—you might say that we are nutritionally *unconscious* if not *comatose*—with little to no understanding of or thought given to what we are eating, why we are eating, or the consequences of that eating.

I will be using the terms *emotional* eating, *mindless* eating, and *promiscuous* eating very often in the pages that follow. In a very simplistic fashion, these descriptors are used interchangeably; however, although these expressions all share many characteristics in common, there are also some distinctions that I would like to clarify. When we eat for emotional reasons, it is often done in a mindless fashion. And when we eat mindlessly, it is frequently accomplished in a promiscuous manner. Whether emotional, mindless or promiscuous or any permutation of the three, we are likely to eat much more than we desire to consume. Under these circumstances, we consume *stealth calories*—calories that we sneak into ourselves when we are not being attentive and that tend to make us gain weight. Although we may experience a wide range of feelings during the actual moment of consumption—ranging from lack of enjoyment to near-orgasmic pleasure as we ravenously down a package of chocolate éclairs—when all is said and done, we are left fatter and often feeling new and different emotions including anger, remorse and guilt.

Emotional eating is defined as eating not driven by physical hunger, but by emotional hunger—usually negative feelings and emotions that beg for relief and comfort (although, at times, positive emotions, including optimism and happiness, that seek reward). In emotional eating, food serves as a drug to take the edge off and soothe our stressed and tense souls. Our emotional state of mind can literally cloud our judgment in a similar manner to alcohol, which can facilitate the consumption of unwanted and unneeded calories. The common emotions that trigger eating are: stress; anxiety; boredom; loneliness; sadness or depression; mood swings; anger; exhaustion; frustration; resentment; disappointment; self-esteem issues; and interpersonal conflicts.

Figuratively speaking, it would seem that what many of us really seek is emotional refuge and respite in the safety, warmth and comfort of our mother's breast, or alternatively, a warm bottle with a nipple on it to nurse our psychic wounds. In other words, we strive for a *transcendental meditative aid*. There was a time during infancy when our mouth served as our pleasure center and the link to the breast or bottle that brought forth our peace, succor, relief, security, and the feeling of control over our environment—not just from hunger and thirst—but also perhaps from fear, distress, loneliness and a myriad of other frightening human emotions. Just because we have advanced chronologically into adulthood does not liberate us from the need for comfort that we received from our nursing and nurturing mothers on such a primal level in our earliest years. On a metaphorical level, at stressful times, what many of us are searching for is the lulling motion of being rocked to sleep, the comfortable feeling of our mother's pulsating heart, the gentle rhythmic shushing sounds emanating from our mother's lips, and her soothing offering of the warm, sweet milk. We may have been weaned a long time ago, but certain situations bring out the presence of our inner infants and beg for primal comfort—food seemingly serving as a substitute or surrogate for the breast or bottle. Some of us reach for a martini, others for a cigarette, others for drugs, still others for comfort food—

all maladaptive behaviors with the intent of orally pacifying our frazzled souls and regaining a state of serenity.

Mindless eating is broadly defined as when we eat without giving thought, focus, and attention to our eating. It involves a lack of self-awareness and self-consciousness that subverts our abilities to control the balance between the pleasure-seeking aspects of eating and the need for restraint. It is typified by eating in a manner that is reflexive, inattentive, unfocused and tuned out to the various dimensions of eating—a perfunctory eating style that does not allow the time to see, smell, hear, touch, and taste our food. It also entails eating rapidly and thoughtlessly with no savoring of the experience nor appreciation of the moment. Whether our mind is temporarily jaded because of emotions and feelings weighing heavily upon us, or whether it is turned off for some other reason, it opens up a huge potential for eating problems. Just as distracted driving causes car accidents, so distractions from mindfulness can cause eating "accidents."

Mindless eating also entails the fact that many of us are just not aware or do not have the knowledge that we are eating "bad" foods. The solution to this is simply acquiring an education on nutrition and eating. Even if we do have a good comprehension of the salutary benefits of healthy eating and conversely, the detrimental effects of unhealthy eating, shifting into a mindless mode can undermine that knowledge.

Promiscuous eating is the wanton, reckless, unselective, casual and indiscriminate consumption of foods without regard to the potential consequences of this "indiscretion." It is characterized by an unhealthy relationship with food and a lack of a long-term commitment to quality foods and eating for the right reasons and in the right manner. Promiscuous eating involves consistently and knowingly making poor food choices that are hazardous to our health and consuming food for purposes other than satisfying genuine hunger. It entails the profligate consumption of food in inappropriate amounts at unsuitable speeds, times and places, often without enjoyment of the eating process. Promiscuous eating often leaves us feeling physically bloated as well as psychologically plagued by guilt, regret, and remorse as an aftermath.

Eating in the manner and style that many of our dogs do—not at all to denigrate the canine species, as I am very fond of Duncan, my English Springer Spaniel—is a simple measure of promiscuous eating. Duncan does not particularly care about what he eats, where he eats, why he eats, when he eats, or how he eats, which is typically like a ravenous wolf. As he gets older, he tends to eat even more voraciously. He sometimes eats so rapidly that he chokes and vomits, and on one or two occasions, has proceeded to eat his own vomit. He is not evolved to the point where he can eat mindfully, and when it comes down to eating behavior, this is the very essence of the difference between lesser evolved animals and human beings.

It might just be that when we stand naked in front of our unforgiving bathroom mirrors we appear "soft in the cage" or perhaps we can grab a handful of flabby flesh around our midriffs. Perhaps the term "roly-poly" comes to mind when we think of an adjective to describe our bodies. Just maybe when we look down we cannot catch a glimpse of our toes without extending our legs forward or sucking in our abdomens. Possibly our pants, skirts or belts are getting a bit on the snug side. Perchance we need to ask the flight attendant for a "seatbelt extender" in order to properly buckle in to the seat of an airplane.

Our best and most honest judge and jury regarding our physical appearance is usually ourselves, with the understanding that our satisfaction with respect to the reflection that we project in a mirror is subject to the vagaries of our own individual sense of body image. We all see the world, and for that matter, ourselves, from the vantage of a unique perspective, and that goes for our body image. There are many whose subjective measure of body image matches an objective assessment, although there are others who have a disconnection or distortion between body image perception and reality, in either direction. If our personal "court of justice" tries and convicts us of a lifestyle "misdemeanor" or lifestyle "felony," it just may be the time to consider a lifestyle audit and then some intelligent and pragmatic strategies to get back into respectable shape.

I do not propose taking medications to this end, although there are specific circumstances under which they may be helpful. I do not recommend bariatric surgery, although there may be no other options for some people. I do not endorse fad diets—ridiculous, outlandish, gimmicky, unbalanced, and unhealthy weight loss schemes are unlikely to cause a meaningful change in our *behavior* and *mindset* that will enable us to keep our weight at an optimal level. What is needed is the establishment of a healthy eating pattern that we can adhere to forever more. As weight gain is usually gradual and insidious, weight loss, accordingly, should be sensible and gradual.

My proposition is to apply the concept of *mindfulness* to eating. Mindfulness is the ability to be present in the moment, purposefully and without judgment. Mindfulness entails an awareness of our body functions, feelings, and consciousness—an attention and a sense of being tuned in to all dimensions of eating. Mindfulness demands education about food and nutrition and behaving in a nutritionally conscientious fashion with the knowledge of the advantageous benefits of healthy eating and the harmful effects of unhealthy eating. Mindfulness necessitates that we understand what we are eating and why we are eating. When brought to the eating domain, mindful eating habits not only demand being mindful when we eat, but also being mindful of being mindful and being mindful of when we are not being mindful.

Cultivating a mindful eating strategy can permit us to become enlightened eaters and commence the journey to liberation from emotional, mindless and promiscuous eating and an unhealthy relationship with food that plays such a major role in engendering weight gain and obesity. It is incumbent upon us to eat for the appropriate reasons. Of equal importance, it behooves us to eat quality and nutritious foods that will provide us with energy and the proper balance of nutrients that will allow us to live a healthy existence.

Our health destiny is—in a significant way—determined by our own food choices. Responsible eating is a lifelong commitment and experiment that should continue to evolve over time if we pursue this journey with a mindful and intelligent attitude. In spite of the convergence of forces that have conspired to promote weight gain and obesity (more about this later), it is still quite possible to have a harmonious relationship with food and maintain a reasonable weight.

The mindful eating strategy that is the premise of this book is geared for all of us: for those who desire to lose weight, for those who desire to maintain a healthy weight, for those who tend to eat for reasons other than genuine hunger, and for those who want to improve their eating habits and nutritional savvy to achieve the healthiest lifestyle possible.

The following is a brief summary of the chapters that follow. Each chapter is sprinkled with quotes from those persons who shared the intimacies of their particular eating behaviors and habits:

THE PROBLEM: UBER-EATING IN THE UNITED STATES OF OBE-SITY explores the reasons underlying the profound overweight and obesity epidemic in America, including our collective emotional state of mind in the new millennium; our increasingly sedentary existence; the relatively inexpensive, addictive, processed foods made ever so accessible by the Industrial Food Complex (IFC); and finally, our culture, where food plays such an enormously prominent role.

THE SKINNY ON WHY WE EAT examines how eating is such a powerful primal gratification—much as sex is—and the various drives and triggers that prompt us to eat. When eating is deconstructed, food going from hand to mouth usually comes down to the following: physical hunger; emotional hunger; recreation and entertainment; opportunity, availability and temptation; accessory eating; social activity; reward; deprivation; boredom; fatigue; drug-induced; ritual; seasonal; hormonal; and habit.

WHAT FOODS TO BE WARY OF: CAVEAT EMPTOR (BUYER BE-WARE) brings to awareness the many unhealthy and unwise food choices that we should make an effort to partake of only on a very sparing basis. The perils of processed foods are discussed in detail and recommendations are made regarding chemical additives, preservatives, artificial colors and dyes, hormones, antibiotics, pesticides, and the often hazardous meat industry. This chapter concludes with a commentary comparing the Industrial Food Complex with the tobacco industry, both responsible for toxic products that have contributed to our poor health.

PSYCHOLOGICAL PERSPECTIVES: THE MIND VIS-À-VIS EAT-ING—BATTLING RAW EMOTIONS WITH FOOD analyzes the mind-body connection, consciousness, and mindfulness vs. mindlessness as it relates to our eating behavior. Classical conditioning, operant conditioning, and Freud's divisions of the psyche are reviewed in order that these perspectives may help us understand and conquer our emotional, mindless, and promiscuous and other dysfunctional eating habits.

SOLUTIONS: CHEW OVER THESE IDEAS provides a practical and pragmatic approach to our eating issues and problems. Necessary tactics, strategies, and solutions to manage our eating problems and to help us achieve our weight loss or weight maintenance goals are enumerated. Cognitive and behavioral principles are delineated and the quotes of many who were interviewed are used to provide reinforcement to the solutions set forth.

RAW FACTS AND TRUTHS succinctly reviews indisputable certainties about weight, body fat distribution, genetics, weight gain, physical fitness, exercising, weight loss programs, and food addiction.

100 VALUABLE NUGGETS AND TIDBITS consists of 100 "pearls" of advice, tricks, suggestions, hints, tips, pointers and simple recipes to facilitate the journey towards health, wellness and a body weight one can be happy with.

My goal for myself as well as for the reader after completing this book is the integration of a mindful philosophy directed towards the act of eating, as captured in the next paragraph. This can be embraced as your own creed or mantra, or used as a general template to be modified to suit your individual needs. Regardless, I feel confident that you, too, will be able to find your way on the journey towards eating in a more mindful, conscious, conscientious and healthy fashion.

I will attempt to eat mindfully and conscientiously, with purpose, attention and focus, recognizing that the primary goal of eating is to fuel myself with quality foods that will promote my health and wellness and avoid preventable diseases. I recognize that eating can be a highly rewarding and pleasurable activity, but as such, has the potential to be abused. I will make every effort to achieve a balance between the pleasure-seeking aspects of eating and the need for disciplined restraint. I will try to avoid eating when I am not hungry and when certain emotional states of mind give me the false sense of hunger. I recognize that this hunger, although perhaps soothed by eating under these circumstances, in reality represents an emotional need that should instead be addressed by an alternative and more appropriate behavior than eating. However, if I must succumb to the desire to eat for emotional reasons, I will make every effort to eat foods that will not cause me to feel guilt or regret, and will promote my good health and wellness.

The Problem

Uber-Eating in the United States of *Obesity*

Caroline, age 53

I really enjoy the taste of food. I get a great deal of comfort and stress relief from eating, especially from rice, pasta, potatoes, and bread. Eating is a means of occupying my hands and satisfying my impulse for oral gratification—especially salty, crispy, crunchy cravings. Out of habit I eat when watching television, when attending Yankee games and when on vacations. A particularly bad habit is eating while driving in the car on long trips. For me, eating fills a void when I'm bored. When I experience insomnia I will go down to the kitchen and eat a few peanut butter and jelly sandwiches in the middle of the night—I realize what a horrid habit that is. My situation is particularly bad in the evening, but well controlled during the day when I am busy and occupied at work. One problem is that I am not mindful of calories, for example the 600-calorie pretzel that I eat at Yankee stadium. Also, I eat way too fast. For me, food is an addiction and I often feel a sense of deprivation that drives my eating.

I am trying to eliminate the late night noshing, focusing on how much better I will feel in the morning. I am trying not to eat those "white" carbohydrates that are my trigger foods for overeating. I am also trying to replace needless eating with other activities. However, the exercise part is a little more challenging, but I am trying to do at least 20 minutes a day of something aerobic.

THE WEAPON OF DESTRUCTION OF THE MASSES

In the 21st century, a combination of factors has created a *perfect storm* to engender weight gain and obesity—the prevalence of which is growing explosively—faster than that of any other public health issue in the history of the USA. Obesity can and will ultimately wreak havoc on our health and lives. Obesity is really just a form of slow, voluntary suicide. While we do not have a great deal of control over that much in our lives, we certainly do have the ability to live a smart lifestyle that avoids malignant and self-destructive behaviors that promote diabetes, hypertension, cardiovascular diseases, cancer, and premature death.

One factor is that our existence has become increasingly stressful, difficult, and messy, and our psychological well being and emotional status can unequivocally affect our eating patterns. We are experiencing a confluence of crises, with our faltering economy, poverty, high unemployment, the banking, mortgage and healthcare and energy meltdowns, global warming, environmental disasters, involvement in several wars, terrorism and post-9/11 paranoia, nuclear threats and fears of weapons of mass destruction, E. Coli and salmonella scares, bedbug infestations, and so on. Secondly, technological advances have supported an increasingly sedentary lifestyle. As mankind has gone from a feral to a domesticated existence and progressive technological advances have made daily living so much easier and so much less physical, we have become the plump, sedentary, and out-of-shape victims of our collective intelligence. Thirdly, the Industrial Food Complex has created a vast array of unhealthy processed foods that are readily available, aggressively marketed and promoted, relatively inexpensive and potentially addictive. Fast foods and many packaged foods—cheap, easy, and a staple of many adults and children—are in this increasingly huge category.

THE ZAFTIG ZEITGEIST

We live in a culture where eating plays an enormously prominent role—I would be so bold as to say that our society is food-obsessed. Food is even an intimate part of our colloquial language. *As easy as pie*, we can go through our entire alphabet—letter by letter—listing food and eating idiomatic expressions. For example, *apple of your eye*, *butter someone up*, *chew the fat*, *drop you like a hot potato*, *eat humble pie*, etc.

Food has transcended its functional capacity to the point where it has been turned into a fetish. This food ethos has contributed to "the problem" by informing our beliefs, customs and practices with respect to eating. In food-centric America, it is very difficult, if not impossible, to avoid exposure to food in the course of our daily activities. With some supermarkets, diners, and 7-Elevens open 24/7, there is no escaping opportunity. Even if we manage to escape from our everyday routine and head away on vacation, we cannot avoid eating as a recreational and leisure activity. In fact, many feel that our vacations give us a sense of eating entitlement and the license to consume with reckless abandon. Food is a key element at weddings, funerals and other rites of passage celebrations including bar and bat mitzvahs, confirmations, graduations, birthdays, etc. Meals are served to us on airplanes, trains, at highway rest stops and five times or more a day on cruises, which are literally eating orgies-on-the-sea. Almost any form of entertainment involves food offered from concession stands—spectator sports, movies, Broadway plays, etc.; at some of these venues food is actually delivered to the spectator who does not even have to arise from his seat to get something to eat! How many of us participate in tailgating parties that go on in the parking lots of every stadium before sporting events?

John, age 26

Eating has become such a hobby—my grandmother's entire life was structured around it. For her, it started with the anticipation, then the meal preparation and finally the consumption. Meals were, for her, the pinnacle of her day.

We don't have to be a spectator in order to be well fed—we can be sports participants as well! On any golf course we will find well-stocked carts being driven around the fairways serving snacks—or if we stop in the club house, we will find foursome after foursome downing cheeseburgers and beers in the break between the front and back nine. Or if we go to any bowling alley, we can observe the consumption of food going on in the middle of play.

Then there is food as entertainment and sport in and of itself—ranging from haute gastronomy with degustation menus to the lowly street stand selling hot dogs. The United States dining scene is a gazillion dollar industry of culinary delights and wonders to gratify our palates—an extensive array of cafes, bistros, brasseries, trattorias, and restaurants. Food enthusiasts can avail themselves of handmade gourmet chocolates, vintage champagnes, imported caviars, artisanal cheeses, heritage turkeys, and so much more. We now have the Food Network and The Cooking Channel to satisfy our insatiable appetite for food programming. Additionally, numerous television and cable shows set in kitchens have flourished dramatically over the last decade and it now appears that *cooking* has achieved the status of being a recognized new genre of entertainment. Food blogging has come of age and is a means of disseminating information on a restaurant's menu, staff, décor, and quality to anyone with an internet connection. Similarly, recipe blogging has come into vogue.

If we take a moment to give it some thought, we may come to the realization that a visit to a restaurant is often replete with certain *absurdities* and *excesses*—we are seated at a table and offered a drink, bread, appetizer, salad and an entrée—literally, often an *insane* amount and variety of food! Do we really want or need to be consuming so massively? And when dinner is completed and the dishes are cleared, we are enticed with dessert, usually a calorie-dense, fat-laden, sugary concoction, so that we end the meal with a sweet taste in our mouths and a final stimulation of our senses. We are not really hungry at that point, but it is tradition, it is tempting, it is entertaining and it is available—in fact, often wheeled to our table for our inspection.

Located ubiquitously throughout America is a glut of fast food chains offering super-sized portions and even drive-through services. On every Main Street, there are an abundance of pizza shops, bagel stores and take-out Chinese food. Virtually every newly constructed gas station has an associated convenience store so that we can fuel our cars and bellies at the same time. We can go to virtually any bookstore and find ample opportunities for food and beverage consumption to accompany our reading consumption. Many a car wash facility now offers food to occupy us while we await the emergence of our shiny vehicles. We can walk down many urban avenues and find carts serving food, into many buildings and find vending machines, and in most any office, doughnuts next to the coffee pot. If we desire to go shopping at the mall and feel a hunger pang, we will find food courts galore.

Our holidays have a very strong emphasis on food and eating—think Thanksgiving feasts; barbeques on Memorial Day, Independence Day and Labor Day; and Valentine's Day, Christmas, Easter and New Year's Eve dinners. Our eating culture literally bombards us with food no matter where we are. Clearly, we need little excuse for eating.

My friend Caesar is originally from Spain, but has lived in the USA for many years and has pointed out to me the difference in attitude many Americans have towards meals and dining as opposed to the Spanish—and for that matter—many other Europeans. The United States food culture is *primarily* about eating and consumption. However, in Spain and much of Europe, the culture is such that the emphasis is on socializing with friends and family—with eating being a *secondary* concern. The other difference between the European and American food cultures is that, for the most part, portions in Europe are small, whereas portions in the United States are often huge. So, not only are there boundless opportunities to consume in the United States, but when we do so, the portions are super-sized with "bigger is better" the seeming American mantra. Unfortunately, the American waistline and derriere are now supersized as well! I guess this explains why when I go to my local sporting goods store to buy a tennis shirt that is an American size *medium*, the tag states European size *large*, and why an American size *small* is a European size *medium*, and so forth.

The obesity epidemic has been "fed" by super-sized American portions served on super-sized plates. Calories add up rapidly when portion sizes are increasingly larger and larger—bagels have become gargantuan and servings of soda in 7-Elevens are 46 ounce sugar-laden monstrosities aptly called *super big gulp*. Many fast food restaurants advertise their portion enormity—Ruby Tuesday's *colossal burger*, Hardee's *thickburgers*, and Burger King's *triple whopper, BK stacker* and *Meat 'Normous breakfast sandwich*, promoted as having a full pound of sausage, bacon, and ham. The Big Texan restaurant in Amarillo, Texas, is famously the "home of the free 72 ounce steak if you can eat it all." Arizona's Heart Attack Grill is a hospital theme restaurant whose menu includes *"single," "double," "triple," and "quadruple bypass"* burgers, ranging from one-half pound to two pounds of beef. Their *"flatliner"* fries are cooked in pure lard. At this restaurant, if you weigh over 350 pounds, you eat for free. Only in America!

If you have the opportunity, watch the entertaining and eye-opening *Super Size Me*—a 2004 documentary directed by Morgan Spurlock in which his diet for a one-month period consisted solely of McDonald's. This movie clearly demonstrates the shocking ill effects of poor food choices on our health and well being.

Because of technological advances, we burn less calories in getting through the course of our day. Our human race is not hard-wired to live a sedentary existence, but is, in fact, designed to be a physically active species. We are not meant to be sitting in cars, trains, and buses, commuting to and from work, perched on our bottoms for lengthy time periods at our desks, peering at our computer monitors, and slouched on the couch for hours every evening watching television. We were originally designed to be chasing our prey through the forest, hustling across the terrain to the nearest river, and hightailing it at top speed to escape the throes of our enemies. However, our collective human brainpower has engendered such profound technological advances that physical activity is no longer a necessity for survival for the vast majority of us. So, although we are programmed at our most fundamental level for physical activity, many of us do not incorporate exercise into our lifestyles and hence pay the price by being overweight, obese and/or physically unfit.

> Many of us have an ingrained, deep-seated discomfort with our bodies. In this technological age, we no longer do much physical work. Our bodies are an inconvenient appendage to our heads. We make our living by reading, writing, speaking, and thinking, but seldom by physical labor. The nature of our work is written on our physiques, and the imprint of our sedentary lifestyle can be read in our posture, gait, and carriage. The physical profile of most middle-age Americans is distressingly similar—necks canted forward, shoulders rounded, abdomens flaccid, appendages skinny and weak . . . Our neglected bodies are repositories for stress, depression, and illness.
>
> Ray Kybartas, *Fitness is Religion—Keep the Faith*

Paralleling technological progress, "advancements" in food science and technology have resulted in an abundance of *processed* and *refined foods* that have increasingly replaced fresh, wholesome, healthy and natural foods in our diet. The Industrial Food Complex is a huge force consisting of such companies as: Kraft, PepsiCo, Nestle, ConAgra, Dean, Sara Lee, General Mills, Kellogg, Unilever, etc. These companies have created a plethora of seductive, addictive, unnatural, unhealthy products containing excessive sugar, fat and salt. Consumption of these products—relatively inexpensive and ubiquitously available—causes our bodies to produce a burst of insulin, which pulls the sugars out of our blood streams and converts them to fats. Before you know it, our blood sugars are low again, which causes us to feel hunger and seek more of these products, perpetuating the addictive cycle and promoting weight gain, obesity, insulin resistance, cardiovascular disease, and more.

The Scripps Research Institute in 2010 conducted a study, published in *Nature Neuroscience* by Paul Kenny and Paul Johnson, essentially showing that compulsive eating shares the same addictive biochemical mechanism as does cocaine and heroin. Using laboratory rats fed high-calorie, high-fat foods, the development of obesity coincided with a progressively deteriorating chemical balance in parts of the brain that deal with reward and pleasure, confirming the addictive nature of junk foods. When offered healthy food alternatives, the rats in the study displayed no interest whatsoever and basically starved. The study concluded that "over-consumption of highly pleasurable food triggers addiction-like neuro-adaptive responses in brain reward circuitries, driving the development of compulsive eating. Common mechanisms may therefore underlie obesity and drug addiction."

Is it any wonder that in less than a few generations, we have gone from the breadlines of the Depression era to wartime food rationing to a situation in which many Americans are overfed yet undernourished on a calorie-rich and nutrient-poor Western diet? We are currently facing a pandemic of obesity among adults and children alike, devastating to both the health of the nation and to our healthcare system. Currently, 75% of the trillions of dollars Americans spend on health care is on four increasingly prevalent diseases: obesity, Type 2 diabetes, cardiovascular disease, and cancer. Many of these diseases are preventable as they are often caused by unhealthy diets, sedentary existences, tobacco and lack of exercise.

Type 2 diabetes mellitus—that due to failure to produce enough insulin or due to insulin-resistance—was formerly known as AODM: Adult Onset Diabetes Mellitus. However, because of the childhood obe-

sity problem and the increasing prevalence of this type of diabetes in children, it had to be renamed!

America is plus-sized with approximately one-third obese and one-third overweight, with only the remaining one-third carrying a healthy weight. Almost 50 million Americans, including 50% of persons older than 60 years of age, suffer with *metabolic syndrome*, defined as having three or more of the following: abdominal obesity; high blood pressure; high serum glucose; high triglycerides; low levels of the "good" cholesterol (HDL); and high levels of the "bad" cholesterol (LDL). It comes as no surprise, then, that some refer to the USA as the *United States of Obesity* and that bariatric (weight loss) surgery has emerged as one of the fastest growing surgical specialties.

CHAPTER 2

The Skinny On Why We Eat

Ruth, age 73

I am a "foodaholic"—addicted to food. Food functions as a pacifier for me. Stress and fatigue drive my eating, as does the scent of a Cinnabon. If I dine out at a restaurant and am unsatisfied with my meal, I feel deprived and the need to binge. My binges last a day or two, but I may have no problem for months at a time. Once I start, I am off the wagon and cannot stop immediately. My key binge food is chocolate. After I open a package, I can't just have a few and need to eat the entire contents, as I am not a controlled eater. With me, it is all or none—that is why I don't keep these types of foods around. I have no respect for overweight people and cannot allow myself to get into that position. My mother had difficulty expressing love, but was able to do so through cooking and not by other means.

Nicole, age 33

My husband is Italian and food, family and eating are really important. We like to cook together, and once I smell good food it triggers my eating. Before I had my kids, I would eat to occupy time, especially during the winter months when I am usually bored. Now that I have children, I am cured of boredom, but I have to eat what I can, while I can, fast, and I often finish off their plates. At a celebration where I give the toast, I end up eating a lot because of the alcohol, the happy atmosphere and the availability of good food—there are lots of intertwined reasons to eat.

Eating and sex are primal gratifications. Our most basic human drive is survival, which is predicated upon having energy (food) to fuel our bodily processes. We have evolved in such a way that the act of fueling, similar to the act of reproducing, is an enjoyable and highly stimulating sensual activity that piques multiple, if not all, our senses, thus driving the behavior. What a clever bait and switch scheme conceived by nature's forces! We consume food seemingly in the pleasurable pursuit of satisfying our hunger, but in reality—determined by this evolutionary sleight of hand—for the purpose of keeping ourselves well fueled and energized.

Imagine if we derived no pleasure from eating and it was done perfunctorily—solely for the purpose of energizing—in similar fashion to when we dispense fuel into our cars, with an emotionally neutral and joyless demeanor. What would happen is we would be doing a lot less eating and obesity would be unheard of; in fact, many would probably be undernourished, which would not benefit survival. Our consumption could probably be limited to a formula containing all the necessary nutrients to sustain a human being that would need to be administered at certain time intervals.

We are hard-wired such that in the absence of fueling beyond a certain time interval we develop the sensation known as hunger, which is an uncomfortable, if not painful, condition that begs quelling. Thus, both the pleasure-seeking behavior (eating for enjoyment) and the displeasure-avoiding behavior (eating to quell hunger) drive our energy consumption, ensuring well-fueled humans and maximizing our potential for survival.

As humans, we are sensual creatures and sensate beings—we enjoy being alive and we relish living. We delight in having our senses tweaked and piqued, which is why so many of us find great enticement in activities such as going to the beach, bicycling, skiing, eating, sex, etc. Perhaps more than any other activity, eating stimulates all of our senses: sight, smell, hearing and touch, in addition to taste.

Because eating is—for many of us, including myself—such a stimulating and pleasurable experience, it is easily and readily liable to over-indulgent behavior. A chemical dependence on food satisfies the criterion for an *addiction*. There are many addictions that humans can succumb to including alcohol, drugs, sex, gambling and eating. Unlike behaviors that involve habits that we can live without, food is unique in that we are all dependent upon it for our survival.

So, we are all food addicts to some extent since without it we would not survive for very long. Although we do not typically develop *tolerance*, in which increasing quantities are needed to result in the same effect, we are all *physically dependent* upon food, such that symptoms of withdrawal will occur if blood levels of glucose fall and engender hunger and cravings. Additionally, because food can stimulate our pleasure centers, it can be viewed as a mood-altering drug possibly leading to compulsive use.

And how easy it is for us to be compulsive abusers—addicts— of food. Food is relatively cheap, it is readily available, and we do not need a dealer or involvement in surreptitious business arrangements or clandestine meetings to get our supply. We don't need to snort it, smoke it, or inject it into our veins. A food addiction is condoned by society and it is often pursued in the company of others. The Industrial Food Complex has created an abundance of highly processed, attractively packaged foods laden with fat, sugar, and salt that are convenient fodder for our addiction. In contrast to the wholesome, slow-digesting, unrefined grains that contain abundant fiber— which slows and regulates glucose absorption and leaves us feeling full and satisfied—these nutritionally-void substances promote addiction. Highly-refined food substances—typified by enriched wheat flour (wheat grain strip mined of the bran and germ)—is a pulverized, super-fine, silky white powder that appears much like cocaine or heroin. Essentially, this pre-chewed, pre-digested, melts-in-your-mouth adult baby food is absorbed very rapidly because of the fiber-stripping and refinement process, much akin to *mainlining* glucose into our bloodstream! And that is just the refined grain component— juice this up with the right combination of sweeteners and fats and you have ingested a *fix*—the physiological result of which is a sugar rush causing a rapid spike in insulin to get the sugar load into our cells. This fix is one that provides a short-lived satisfaction that begs the use of more and more. If this eating behavior is maintained, it can damage our system that metabolizes carbohydrates and sugars, with the possibility of diabetes ensuing.

So why is it that so many of us have an unhealthy and abusive relationship with food, but not with other absolute necessities of life such as air and water? You do not see too many compulsive air abusers who trek up mountains and inhale away incessantly as they take in the beautiful vistas or those who purposely get on a treadmill to get so winded so that they can suck in extra air! (It is nice, though, to go to yoga class and focus on our breathing and make it foreground instead of background, or after a rainstorm, go outside and take deep inhalations of the rarefied, sweet air.) And water—more so than food, we are so dependent upon it that within a few days of its absence we would die—is rarely abused!

Many things in life, then, are *not so good with as they are bad without*. Air and water satisfy this concept—when we have a ready supply of air and water, we really do not give them a second thought, but if we are in a situation where we are lacking either—say trapped in a cave with minimal oxygen or after a long run in the heat of the summer without any water supply—they become of critical importance. However, for many people, food is different—it is clearly *bad without* as hunger is a kind of pain that we seek to quell, but it is equally *good with*, food having a wonderful ability to tweak the pleasure centers of our brain.

In spite of food being the "addictive" substance that it is, one in three Americans is able to maintain a stable and healthy weight by striking a balance between the potential for overeating and the need for disciplined restraint. A healthy and appropriate relationship with food is of great importance in helping promote this balance. Before putting any food substance into our mouths, we need to be mindful of the following questions: *Is this item something that we want to place into our physical selves? Do we want this to actually become us—to be integrated into our beings? What exactly are we putting in our mouths? What is its provenance (origin/source)? Why are we consuming it? Where are we pursuing this activity? When are we eating? How are we eating? How much are we eating?*

Two out of three Americans are overweight or obese. The drives to eat are the ability for food intake to satisfy hunger and the pleasure derived from eating, in addition to the short-term benefits seemingly derived from eating for emotional reasons. Overeating may result from an abnormal inability to satisfy hunger, eating for psycho-emotional reasons, or from excessive pleasure seeking behavior. In this regard, there are gourmand-epicurean-foodies who simply love to eat and engage in extreme gustatory indulgences. The collateral effect of the pursuit of such earthly delights, regardless of the reason, is the consumption of too many calories.

There is a bell curve for the amount of food necessary to satisfy our hunger—for some, it takes a small volume of food, but others have a seemingly insatiable appetite (myself included in this latter category). Our hunger is certainly not a constant from moment to moment and can vary substantially depending upon external and internal influences. Fluctuating hormone levels in women can profoundly affect hunger, with many women reporting a "ravenous" appetite in the week or so before menstruation as well as accompanying pregnancy. Additionally, the variable amount of sunlight in a day based upon the seasons can impact our hunger, with many people in Northern hemispheres reporting an increased appetite during the shorter days of the winter months. This is probably multi-factorial, with biochemical triggers resulting from the decreased light stimulation and may be related to the "hibernation mode" of winter. This can help explain the seasonal weight gain that many of us experience over the autumn and winter months and the shedding of that weight in the spring and summer months.

For many of us, excess caloric consumption is driven simply by ignorance regarding nutrition, resulting in eating the wrong foods. For some of us, it is just a question of not being mindful to know when to stop eating—when enough is enough. Mindfulness, education, nutritional conscientiousness and some savvy regarding eating can rapidly correct this and provide us with the knowledge and wisdom to rectify these remediable issues.

Eating should be a *pleasure*-driven and not a *pain*-driven human behavior. Pain-driven eating occurs when negative emotions are quelled by eating—the motivation to eat bearing absolutely no relationship to hunger—the food consumption providing comfort and compensation for fatigue from lack of sleep, stress, mood swings, loneliness, depression, boredom, etc. When eating for such reasons becomes an ingrained habit, an unhealthy relationship with food has been fostered. Any altered state of consciousness can lead to such mindless "hypnotic autopilot eating" patterns. Eating can sometimes be driven by the need for immediate gratification or as a form of self-loathing and self-abusive behavior. Sometimes the driving factor for consumption is the use of drugs including alcohol or marijuana.

In the next few pages, I will attempt to systematically enumerate the variety of different forces that drive our eating behavior. This system is somewhat arbitrary as all classification systems are, given that there is overlap among the different reasons. However imperfect, this system—derived from what I have learned after interviewing many people about what triggers their eating—hopefully will help explain the various motivations for our eating behavior, particularly when we eat when not hungry. It is often this eating when not hungry that contributes to the highly prevalent problem of either being overweight or obese. The motivation that prompts many of us to eat can involve several of the following types of eating behaviors acting at the same time:

Hunger eating: We were designed to experience hunger when our bodies demand caloric replenishment and the feeling of satiety when we are sated, and it is ultimately this hunger that drives our eating and not the clock. We need energy and sustenance in the form of calories and although our culture has created the sanctioned-by-society-breakfast-lunch-dinner-three-meal-a-day-plan, when you give it some thought, it is really quite contrived.

The physiological basis for eating—what precisely it is that functions to cause us to experience hunger and seek food—is complex and multi-factorial. Two hormones, *leptin* and *ghrelin*, appear to play important roles. Leptin, a satiety hormone, is produced by fat cells and gives the message to the brain to reduce appetite. When we are in need of energy, leptin levels drop, resulting in appetite stimulation. Ghrelin (Growth *h*ormone *rel*easing plus the word *in*), is a circulating hunger hormone secreted primarily by the stomach and pancreas that functions as an appetite stimulant. Ghrelin levels increase prior to eating and decrease after consumption.

Marcos, age 30

I eat only for necessity, not for enjoyment. I hate the feeling of being full—it makes me unproductive and keeps me from doing the things that I like to do. I saw a lot of hunger when I grew up in the Dominican Republic, and the food culture in the United States was shocking to me when I first came here.

Hobby/recreational/entertainment eating: Bon Appétit! Eating has become much more than the simple ingestion of calories to provide the energy and nutrients necessary for survival. Eating is downright enjoyable and piques and stimulates *all* of our senses; there are few among us who do not seek and relish the pleasure and gustatory titillation that eating provides. Some of us love the sensation and sound of food crunching between our teeth or melting on our tongues; others delight in the actual process of chewing; still others enjoy the feel of food gliding down our throats. Then, of course, there are the tantalizing aromas and the often sheer artistry of a beautifully-prepared meal.

That being said, there are some for whom eating is a mundane and perfunctory activity—those who truly *eat to live*. But there are many foodie-epicurean-gourmand-sybarite types who absolutely adore eating, and for whom eating can be considered a genuine hobby, recreational activity, and form of entertainment—those who *live to eat*. In America, there is ample opportunity for eating as sport, with an abundance of superlative restaurants serving every imaginable ethnicity of food and appealing to every conceivable palate. There are many who not only enjoy the cooking and preparation of anything from a simple dish to haute cuisine, but equally relish the consumption of their creations.

Mitchell, age 52

I cook incredible meals and tend to binge on them.

Ted, age 47

I love the sensation of different tastes and a broad spectrum of flavors—I cannot be fulfilled with one flavor on my plate and am in search of and need multiple flavors to be satisfied.

Jackie, age 50

My husband loves to cook and is insulted if I don't eat.

Opportunistic eating: *Build it and they shall come; leave it out and it shall be devoured.*

Unexpected and unanticipated food opportunity can ambush our good intentions. When *opportunity* coexists with *desire*, eating will inevitably occur. Even if opportunity exists without desire, eating often seems to be the consequence. When we are at work and there is a box of enticing doughnuts available and accessible, even if we are not hungry, it will take some degree of willpower for us to avoid the temptation to indulge—if we do partake, we often feel that we are innocent victims of circumstances beyond our control.

Opportunity is a potent force driving our eating—this is recognized and understood by many of us and often managed by those of us who are concerned with our weight and fitness, by *subverting* opportunity. Opportunity can be undermined simply by not having tempting and fattening foods available in our homes; or alternatively, keeping them relatively inaccessible, for example, high up on a top shelf in the pantry. Human nature being what it is—with a tendency towards gravitating towards the path of least resistance—causes us to be less inclined to eat something if it is not readily available, and particularly if access is difficult, especially when hunger is not the motivating force. The adage about the low hanging fruit getting picked before the high hanging fruit is very relevant here.

Ken, age 48

Where I go astray is on the road, because I'm in sales and many of my clients are 7-Elevens, Quick Checks, and Mom and Pop type stores. I am constantly being offered food—a doughnut here, a sandwich there, etc.—I have a great appetite, love to eat and don't want to insult my clients. Stress doesn't help the matter as I have had a number of jobs in the last few years, some in companies that have gone out of business. I have gained 15 lbs or so; I just eat too much volume—even if I'm eating healthy foods, I overdo it. I lack portion control and am less active than I used to be, which doesn't help. I once went to Jamaica with my wife on vacation and in one week, because of the constant availability of food and my bingeing, I gained 10 lbs! That's the truth! For breakfast this morning I had two large bagels with peanut butter and six cups of coffee.

Isabelle, age 10
When opportunity knocks at the door, I answer it.

Jacqueline, age 19
I eat when I am offered food. Late at night, I often join my friends at the diner for a cup of coffee. What happens is that I end up eating a whole meal even though I am not hungry.

Temptation eating: We can be watching television and see a food commercial that entices us to seek out that food or an alternative, even if we are not hungry. Food was not on our mind, but just the sight of it is enough to drive desire. Even merely reading about eating, or talking about it, or even thinking about it can tempt us—as can the actual sight and scent of food and beverage items. This can happen if we are walking in our neighborhood on a nice summer day and breathe in the aroma of hamburgers being barbecued—that smell is all it takes to whet our appetites and desires to find a hamburger pronto! The same holds true for walking through a bakery and having our olfactory sense titillated by the scent of warm, sweet, buttery cookies. The bottom line is that any form of sensory stimulation brought upon by food or any abstraction of food is simply enough to entice us to eat, regardless of our hunger status.

After lunch on a Sunday on a bitter winter day, I was lying on the couch relaxing in the family room, enjoying The New York Times. I had eaten a fine meal and was quite satisfied. In the kitchen, adjacent to the family room, my wife was cooking up some organic potato latkes for my daughters. The delectable aroma that wafted into the family room was incredibly tempting and in fact, irresistible! All I wanted was a little taste, just to quell my craving. But alas, there was not a crumb left by the time I moseyed into the kitchen. All I had wanted was a bite of these seasoned, aromatic potatoes. Frustrated, I foraged and found some leftover whole wheat linguini in the refrigerator, sprinkled it with garlic salt, and heated it up in the microwave. That did the trick . . . the only problem was that the trick was on me because I wasn't really hungry!

Isabelle, age 10

When I hear the sound of food being eaten, it makes me hungry.

Danielle, age 18

When I join my friends for dinner and see food, I get hungry. Advertisements for food get me hungry—fast food, Applebees, IHOP, barbequed rib commercials. Watching the Food Channel makes me hungry. If I am watching a movie and the characters are eating, I get hungry. Buffets make me eat a lot. I have the habit of always eating after school even if I'm not hungry. I eat leftovers until they are finished because I want to get rid of them. I eat when watching television on my computer so I have something to hold and occupy my hands. When sad, I lose my appetite. When busy, I don't think about eating. If I overeat, my stomach hurts and I stop, feeling very guilty. I say I'll diet tomorrow, but never do; I say I will lift weights and run on the treadmill tomorrow, but never do.

Jackie, age 50

I see my kids eating and this triggers my desire to eat.

Accessory eating: This is eating that occurs *incidental* to another activity. As cuff links are an accessory to a dress shirt, eating is often an accessory to many spectator activities including watching television, movies, theatre or ballgames. It is not that we are hungry; it is just that eating under these circumstances can be considered part of the whole process of enjoyment and entertainment. Popcorn, candy and soda are accessory to movies; hot dogs and cracker jacks to the ballpark; and cotton candy to the state fair.

My wife, for instance, cannot sit in front of the television without eating. It is virtually a reflex response for her as well as many a couch potato. Turn on the television—get a snack to complement the process. Another name for this type of food consumption is *reflexive* eating, a form of classical conditioning. Fortunately, my wife is very slim, so her media munchies don't really affect her weight the way it would for many of us.

Liesel, age 53

I eat to live and not vice-versa; I am usually not very hungry. But when the TV is on I am compelled to eat candy, peanuts, raisins, sweets and salts. I crave eating licorice—it is very complicated, but I associate eating licorice with relaxing—because I know that I will be eating it when relaxing, I am drawn to it. Licorice for me is a metaphor for relaxation.

Ted, age 47

Watching movies at home triggers a "snack response"—popcorn, chips, soda, chocolate, breadsticks—it's all about entertainment.

Gwen, age 63

When talking on the telephone, I will eat ice cream or any food available.

Mitchell, age 52

I find it comforting to eat when watching television, like popcorn and a slushy at the movies or smoking and coffee fifty years ago. Snacks and television/movies seem to go together. When I watch television, I enjoy sugary products like cookies and ice cream. I have a snack room at work and can't sit at my desk without eating—especially salty snacks like pretzels and chips—they are the "calmers of my mind."

George, age 53

My ballgame story: I went to a Met game with a friend. There were two strangers sitting in front of us in the box seats. Every couple of innings, my friend and I would leave to buy food, always asking our box mates if they wanted anything and they always refused. Finally, I said to them, "I hate people who only eat when they are hungry"!

Rachel, age 48

When watching television or a movie, I expect to be entertained, and so much of eating is for entertainment.

Bruce, age 54

Reading is my downfall. I am in the habit of eating easy foods like peanuts, chips, and cookies while I'm reading the newspaper. If I haven't finished the paper but have finished the food, I must get more food. I'm usually pretty good during the week, but fall apart on weekends when I'm at home and need to read a lot for school.

Social eating: *No man is an island* and most of us humans, in fact, are rather social creatures. We are often faced with a variety of social situations in which eating is a primary focus. Under the circumstances where other members of the group are eating, we often eat to conform to the will of the group, since we desire to fit in and do not want to be viewed as unsociable. Food is a key element at social events such as weddings, funerals and other rite of passage celebrations including bar/bat mitzvahs, confirmations, graduations, birthdays, etc. Many business enterprises are based upon relationships and connections that are built around meals at restaurants, just as personal relationships often are. "Let's do lunch" often equates to "let's do business." For example, lunch is frequently used as the "calling card" for pharmaceutical representatives to gain a foothold into many medical offices, including my own.

Jennifer, age 40

To me, socializing means eating.

Anne, age 47

I am a big social eater, which is very similar to being a social smoker. I eat out a lot and get excited and pumped about food. I love going to Grand Lux Cafe to enjoy a good meal. I am a big coffee drinker, and coffee begs for food to accompany it.

Leah, age 35

I do not have a love affair with food but do love restaurants. Others may dance or play tennis, but my socializing revolves around food. All of my celebrations involve food. If I see dish that I love, even if not hungry, it has a Pavlovian effect on me.

Reward eating: This type of eating occurs either as a means of remuneration for achieving some sort of accomplishment or, alternatively, as a compensation for some of the perceived difficulties and hardships of our daily existences. For example, we just received a nice raise in salary at work, so we go celebrate with a large piece of cake or an ice cream sundae.

Warren, age 47

It is a reward thing for me—after a long day at work, lots of stress and a long commute home—I feel that I owe myself. Cake is my weakness—I don't eat it all at once, but once started, have continued cravings for it and will need to continue eating it until it is consumed and until I eventually get sick of it—it is like a gambling addiction. I do have long periods of time in which I do not eat cake, and when "clean" I have absolutely no urge for it and the thought of it can be revolting.

Richard, age 51

"Food is love and I need hugs." I'm a happy eater, eating when I get in a good mood. Food is a reward after a difficult presentation. When stressed from work I lose my appetite. I don't eat out of nervousness when preparing a talk or helping my daughter prepare a speech, but after, I eat like a horse—there literally is not enough food in the house. I cannot walk away from food and love to eat good quality food. The quantity I eat is out of control—even though I eat healthy, low-fat, low-carbohydrate foods, my stomach is so stretched out that to feel full, I need to eat a "psychotic" quantity. My wife says I am a dog and will eat anything; I am truly a garbage disposal.

Ted, age 47

After sex, I feel like I burned calories and deserve replenishment.

Deprivation eating: A sense of deprivation can drive our eating behavior. Feeling needy because of a lack of fulfillment or on the basis of feeling cheated out of what we feel should be our due, can provoke eating. Under these circumstances, we are using the psychological defense mechanism of *sublimation*, using food as a surrogate means of filling a void in our lives. Essentially, a lack of fulfillment pushes us to fill our stomachs. Unfortunately, it is not very effective and can result in unwanted weight gain.

Alicia, age 54

I use eating, yoga and meditation to fill a void, as others might use alcohol, cigarettes and hobbies.

Boredom eating: Many of us use eating as an *activity*—something to do. We enjoy staying occupied and productive and find that when we have nothing much to do, eating can serve the purpose of keeping our hands occupied and our time utilized. Eating piques us with a barrage of multi-sensory stimulation: creamy, crispy, grainy, hot, cold, crunchy, tingly, sweet, spicy, bitter, salty, aromatic, etc. Had we been engaged and absorbed in another matter, the thought of eating would never have entered our minds. We humans need to *pass time* productively and boredom-driven eating does not qualify for constructive time usage and should always be considered a self-destructive *pastime*.

Sheila, age 62

Boredom makes me eat. I get home from mahjong at 11PM, and am not even hungry, but go for the 100-calorie cookie packs. My problem is that I end up eating 6 bags.

Vittoria, age 50

I eat when bored at work—chips, yogurt, chocolate—I do not even think about eating if busy and not bored.

Nancy, age 28

I eat on weekends when I am home, when I am bored, inactive and have nothing to do, primarily to keep myself occupied during downtimes. I also eat while watching TV and on the computer. I like pepperoni, cheese, trail mix, ice cream—I just don't know how to eat healthy and I have gained 40 lbs in 5 years. I eat the wrong things for the wrong reasons. I sometimes feel guilt or regret, especially when my stomach feels heavy.

Justine, age 27

Boredom prompts me to eat. I was unemployed for 8 months and gained 10 lbs. When I have nothing to do, I eat—especially cheese and cookies. Now that I am employed, it is less of an issue.

Fatigue eating: Eating can serve as a substitute for many activities, one of them being sleep. I find that when I am physically and mentally exhausted, in a disassociated "zombie"-type state, I often seek refuge in the refrigerator or pantry in spite of not being the least bit hungry. It seems that this FATigue—an altered state of mind and body—would best be served by seeking refuge in my bed, but mindless food foraging serves as a surrogate activity.

There appears to be a physiological basis for this fatigue-driven eating. Sleep deprivation or the need for sleep results in decreased levels of *leptin*, our chemical appetite suppressant, and increased levels of *ghrelin*, our appetite stimulant, in addition to increased levels of *cortisol*, one of the stress hormones. This sleep-deprived change of our internal chemical milieu can drive our eating.

Drug-induced eating: I include alcohol and marijuana under this category, although other psychopharmacological medications can also affect eating behavior. Alcohol is a depressant that can suppress certain inhibitory functions of the brain, including our ability to have self-control over our eating—our tighter rein over our behavior is loosened up a bit. If we are stone cold sober, it is much more likely that we will exercise sobriety with respect to our eating behavior. Additionally, the load of liquid carbohydrates in the alcoholic beverage—whether it is wine, beer or hard liquor—is quickly absorbed, causing a rapid rise in blood sugar. This triggers the release of insulin that gets the glucose into our cells. As glucose levels drop, hunger receptors are thus stimulated, driving our appetites. Also, the aftermath of the hangover that may ensue from over-consumption of alcohol may include overeating high calorie, fattening foods. Regarding the marijuana munchies, it seems that chemicals known as *endocannabinoids* activate receptors in the hypothalamus of the brain that stimulate the desire to eat.

Justin, age 35

When stressed, I sometimes have a few alcoholic beverages. Sometimes on the weekend I may drink too much and when I am hung over, I need a fattening breakfast, like a bacon and cheese sandwich. This leads to a very bad cycle for me.

Ritual/religious/holiday/tradition eating: Many religions have ceremonies or rituals that involve eating (and interestingly, fasting, as well)—Catholic communions, Jewish Passover Seders, etc. Then there is the typical holiday eating associated with such celebrations as Independence Day, Thanksgiving, Valentine's Day and New Year's Eve.

Emotional eating: We are humans and are extremely emotional creatures and it these highly evolved feelings that are one of the key features that separate us from other members of the animal kingdom. We bring our emotions to every situation that we encounter, and on a certain level we are all emotional eaters since we all bring our emotions "to the plate" in this sense. It is literally impossible to separate emotions from eating and with this in mind, it becomes easier to understand how our emotions can engender dysfunctional eating patterns. There are wide ranges of emotions that can trigger eating. Exhaustion, stress, boredom, anxiety, anger, loneliness, sadness, depression, frustration, resentment, disappointment, issues of self-esteem, and interpersonal conflicts are some of the *negative* emotions that can drive eating. *Positive* emotions including hopefulness, happiness and confidence can also spark emotional eating. In general, it appears that negative emotions demand neutralizing and positive emotions fuel our passion for eating. There are many among us who use food as a refuge from negative emotions, and for whom food serves as both a "friend" and "therapist," but there are some of us who turn off from eating under the same circumstances. Thus, there is a wide range of eating responses to emotions and all of us "metabolize" our feelings differently.

Christine, age 51

I eat because of "nerves"—when I have anxiety, but also when I am confused, frustrated, upset, unfocused, or bored. I worry mostly about financial issues—I have an older son with medical problems and other kids to raise, an old house that I can barely take care of and an ex-husband who is a nightmare. I worry about being alone. I am flying by the seat of my pants and am very disgusted. I hate my life and am living just because I have kids. I eat carbohydrates and fats: pasta, macaroni and cheese, French fries—I get temporary comfort and then am disgusted with myself.

Camille, age 38

I am a "happy eater" at which time I will have a Skinny Cow ice cream, some chocolate or maybe one Oreo cookie. When stressed, down, or depressed, I lose my appetite and pull into my shell and read.

Rachel, age 48

When I am stressed, upset, or bored I will eat cookies. What I do is just eat a few, but then I go back and eat a few more, and then I go back and eat a few more until I bang my head and say "enough." I probably get no relief—it is "useless" with a very short-lived compensation and I feel very guilty.

Jane, age 58

I eat when I am pissed and frustrated or upset because somebody said something to me and I have not been able to deal with it. I am not hungry and I don't enjoy the pasta, chocolate candy or chocolate milk that I down. I feel horrible and bloated after and the guilt is really bad and sometimes causes me to spit out what I am eating. I get very angry with myself and compensate by eating less after and exercising more. Sometimes after work I will eat half a large bag of chips; I will then skip dinner.

Rebecca, age 32

I do "emotional starvation." I only really eat when I am very happy—and at those times a lot of junk food, and much more quantity than normal—this is when food appeals to me and when I gain weight. Normally I have to force myself to eat.

Chris, age 53

Depression and boredom demand cookies, cake and chocolate. I get no real relief, but it's something to do. I have "justifiable" guilt, meaning guilt that I can justify and rationalize. I will compensate by stopping this behavior and exercising more.

Alicia, age 54

Anger, stress, and boredom drive my eating. I tend to eat on the basis of anger and stress on weekdays and because of boredom on weekends. Salt is my addiction. In particular, holiday family get-togethers precipitate deep-seated emotions and tend to drive my overeating for days and days after.

Amanda, age 35

Stress and exhaustion, also happiness, sadness, depression and being upset drive my eating. Yesterday I had a particularly stressful and exhausting day. On my commute home, I anticipated eating. I came in the door to my home, dropped my purse and went right to the fridge, not even bothering to heat up the food. I stuffed my face while talking on the phone to my mother. I enjoyed it and did not regret it. I go for pasta, chocolate, and cheese. This does not seem to be a problem on weekends. After my separation, I ate only "carbs" and junk—cocoa puffs for breakfast, lunch and dinner for three months.

> **Stress eating:** Stress seems to be our most compelling emotional drive to eat, second only to hunger. It is the rare person who does not lead a stressful existence. Stress seems to pummel our souls and eating serves as a mechanism to sooth our beaten-up inner beings— a means of distracting us from our troubles and escaping from the real-life problems and unpleasant aspects of our daily lives. Life can oftentimes be very tough and food can provide an immediate source of comfort and relief, just as a cigarette can to a smoker or alcohol to a drinker. Many of us, particularly after a very stressful day, head straight for the refrigerator after arriving home from work, seeking solace, refuge and sanctuary.

Monique, age 41

Stress and nervousness cause me to eat sweets, especially chocolate and sweet coffee. I do nervous drawing, sketching and doodling as well. If something is on my mind, I will eat an excessive amount of fruit—perhaps 3-5 pieces after 10PM. I enjoy the act of chewing food when I need to think things out and sort out finances. For example, my husband is diabetic, I worry about paying for college for my son who is a high school senior, my parents need medicines, my dad has colon cancer, my mom is paralyzed, our tenant doesn't pay rent. I feel relief, but guilty, and I think tomorrow will be better, but tomorrow brings another stress—it's never-ending.

Katherine, age 56

I am an extremely selective, very picky vegetarian who does not fulfill cravings randomly. I tend to overeat when in social situations. I go out to dinner with friends three or four times a week—in a restaurant environment it is much harder to "tow the line." Nothing makes me happier than a good meal and companionship. My job used to be a respite for me; because of changes due to a merger, it is no longer a source of fulfillment. My home life is very stressful—my kids are "off the grid" and I haven't been involved in a relationship in a long time. I am always at my thinnest when I have a man in my life. My heavier weight directly correlates with my hating my job, lack of a relationship, and the fact that both my kids are in severe distress. My daughter dropped out of college with seven courses to go. My son is aggressive and verbally abusive. So, I have stress at work and aggravation at home. My girl-friend calls and suggests that we meet at the Cheesecake Factory. This serves as a lit-tle oasis from the stress of my life. Food provides me with gratification when nothing else is fulfilling. When my head is not in a good place, I tend to eat unhealthy, bad foods. I feel guilt and remorse, say I'll never do it again, but do it again and again. I even bought a Pilates machine.

As I learned from some of those I interviewed, even "pre-stress," defined as the stress that arises from anticipation of stress, can drive eating.

Lauren, age 34

I eat when I feel stress coming on—when I am "pre-stressed"—for example, when I know in advance that I will have to sit in traffic for 2 hours. I want a combination of sweet and salty, so I buy a dried fruit and nut package. I eat the entire package while driving, 90 grams of fat—over 800 calories from the fat alone! After, I feel dis-gusted and guilty and rationalize it by thinking of the protein and fruit. I compen-sate by eating a smaller dinner. Another example is when I am late getting home and I know my kids will be eating junk and not a healthy meal—because I feel the stress coming on, I am compelled to consume.

Interestingly, it seems that when we eat for negative emotional reasons we tend to gravitate to unhealthy "bad" foods—it would ap-pear that we desire the kind of foods that will match the emotion driving the eating. Self-destructive emotions beg for self-destructive eating behaviors and self-destructive foods.

Susan, age 45

I eat when I am exhausted, stressed or aggravated—most often regarding finances—I'm in charge of everything at home, even making my husband's doctor appointments and buying all his clothes. I go for breads, cheese and crackers and occasionally chocolate. When stressed, I will change my dinner from something healthy and more involved to something quick, easy and less healthy like pasta with sauce and bread. I do get relief while eating, but probably not after and experience a kind of guilt. I say to myself: "I'm going to stop eating in response to stress"; "I'm going to work on not being stressed." These promises are typically kept for a few days.

Also of importance is that when we seek relief from stress by eating, although we may relieve the stress, we also run the risk of engendering new emotions including guilt, regret and shame, which are equally as stressful to us as the original stress that brought upon the eating. So, the *primary stress* elicits eating that then induces secondary stress that may provoke further eating—this is a vicious cycle that is worth steering clear of!

Mitchell, age 52

Stress and idleness are the biggest drivers of my eating when not hungry. The stress is alleviated, but remorse and guilt undo the benefit; essentially, I have traded one emotion for another. I feel bad after overeating; my body is unhappy and my mind is unhappy. I especially feel guilty when eating garbage as opposed to healthy foods.

Nora, age 60

Stress eating occurs when I am overwhelmed—I'll eat anything that doesn't eat me first! For example, a cardiac arrest occurred in our medical office requiring CPR done by the EMTs. I stopped on my way home and bought a bag of chips and started eating in the car. Afterwards, I am guilty thinking about how many calories I have consumed, but the guilt causes me to eat even more!

Bruce, age 54

When stressed, I seek high-fat, high-salt products such as chips, Reese's peanut butter chocolate, ice cream, and Cheez Doodles. I get temporary relief but then experience stress from my eating behavior. I will compensate via exercise and eating well the next day.

It is important to point out that although stress is a huge trigger for eating for many of us, some of us respond in a diametrically opposite way by losing our appetites when confronted with the pressures and tensions of life. Instead of eating food, it would seem that some of us eat our "body parts."

Liesel, age 53

When stressed, the sight of food sickens me. For example, if I am in the supermarket and need to get home quickly to get the kids off the bus, unpack the groceries, prepare dinner, etc., I get nauseated. When I go food shopping, I am less hungry than any other day. When stressed, I "eat my stomach out."

Vittoria, age 50

When stressed, I do not eat food—I eat my cuticles until they bleed.

Kirsten, age 31

Eating is my last priority when stressed.

And there are those who have different eating responses in accordance with the type and degree of stress:

Maria, age 24

When I experience "personal stress" such as when emotionally distraught from having my heart broken, I do not eat at all. However, if it is work stress, for example, when I feel I hate my job, I eat.

Anne, age 47

When under severe stress, for example, a death in family, I stop eating; but when under day-to-day stress I am driven to eat junk food such as Pop Tarts.

Vanessa, age 47

The stress of my daily existence drives my eating. I will eat anything, but go for crunchy, sweet carbohydrates. I feel some relief, scold myself, but don't feel guilty. When I am hugely stressed, for example—when my mom was diagnosed with cancer—I stop eating completely.

There is a biochemical explanation for stress eating. The adrenal gland hormone *cortisol*—released in response to stress—can stimulate our appetites and cravings for sugar, and cause fat storage, thereby promoting weight gain and obesity. This is the very reason people on corticosteroid medications tend to have enormous appetites, gain weight and have a central distribution of body fat known as centripetal obesity. Cortisol also functions to reduce leptin, further stimulating our appetites. Additionally, the consumption of certain foods, especially those containing sugar and fat, can cause release of *endorphins* that are powerful morphine-like chemicals with pain-relieving properties. Is it any wonder that for many, food serves as a sedative? It is of great interest to note that exercise can release prodigious amounts of these endorphins, so better to head to the gym than the fridge when stressed!

Magdalene, age 56

I am on prednisone intermittently to help manage my rheumatoid arthritis. When I am on the steroids, I have no satiation and always gain weight.

Jackie, age 50

I am a stress eater. My father recently died, I take care of three kids, two dogs, and my mother. For example, the other night my mother fell and I had to take her to the emergency room. I came home after midnight and had two pieces of chocolate cake. It provided slight relief, but afterwards I asked myself why I did it and I hate myself for it. It becomes a vicious cycle.

Jill, age 46

I work as an operating room nurse in a hospital. After an emotionally stressful day, while driving home, I plan and anticipate my eating, looking forward to it. Lying prone on the couch, while watching mindless TV like Oprah, I eat popcorn or chips and dip. I end up doing this two or three times a week. I have no regrets even though I know how bad it is. It is a drug for me, numbing everything.

Seasonal eating: For many of us, winter is the season for weight gain and, conversely, summer the season for weight loss. There seem to be a number of very valid explanations for this phenomenon. It seems to start with Halloween sweets, continue with Thanksgiving feasts, and is sustained with the December holidays with all of the many opportunities for parties and excessive eating. *Hiver*, which is the French word for winter, also means hibernation—many of us may experience a vestige of the hibernation mode in which we are impelled by a biological imperative to eat more, perhaps on a biochemical basis having to do with decreased daylight exposure. The cold temperature itself seems to foster a foraging behavior for many of us.

Additionally, in winter, because of weather constraints, we tend to be more housebound with more opportunity for boredom eating and less distractions from eating. In winter, we have less opportunity for outdoor exercise and activities and less availability of healthier fresh fruit and vegetables that are more readily available in summer. Unhealthier, "heavier" comfort foods, including stews, creamy soups and starches, seem to be the antidote for cold weather and darkness.

Perhaps *seasonal affective disorder*—the winter-related gloom experienced by many of us, including myself—influences our eating behavior by toying with our emotions. Finally, many seem just to care less about their physical appearance during those times of the year when they are less likely to need to get into shorts or a bathing suit, so are less attentive to their eating.

Talia, age 56

In summer, I eat lighter and healthier, more fruits and salads; from Halloween to New Years, I gain weight with all the socializing. My winter comfort foods are breads, pastas and other carbohydrates.

Leah, age 35

During winter, I eat much more than I do so in summer. It's about being stuck indoors and the cold, dark and gloom when I wake up and return from work. I seek comfort foods including starches, hearty stews and heavy wines like cabernets. Also, I don't really care about how I look in bikinis and shorts since it is winter. During the summer because it is hot, I consume less calories, drink lighter white wines like Sauvignon Blancs and am much more concerned about my appearance.

Chris, age 53

Winters are way worse in terms of my eating. I can't exercise the way I want to and end up working out in my humid basement, which I do not enjoy. I hate awakening in the dark and cold and arriving home in the dark and cold.

Kerrie, age 46

During summer, I do less eating and more grilling, which is a healthier way of preparing meats. During winter, I'm stuck in the house, it's way too cold and I watch more movies which means more eating, especially cookies.

Habit eating: We are humans and are very much creatures of habit. Habits occur when behaviors are repeated until they are reinforced and gain traction. For many of us, eating while watching television, a DVD, or sporting events is a habit, as is eating while talking on the telephone or surfing the internet. Many of us have developed the habit of eating upon entrance into our homes, where we walk directly to the kitchen and go on a food rampage; some of us eat when our children arrive home from school in mid-afternoon; and a considerable number of us habitually eat while preparing dinner.

Kyle, age 44

When in New York City, I must have 2 "dirty water dogs"—those hot dogs sold by the vendors from the pushcarts.

Hormonal eating: Many of the women I interviewed related that in the week or so prior to menstruation, they experience an augmented appetite and cravings for certain foods, particularly salts. This is similar to how pregnancy affects appetite and hunger. The consensus seems to be a ravenous appetite with cravings for carbohydrates and salt.

Jennifer, age 40

Being pregnant gives me the license to eat whatever and however much I want.

CHAPTER 3

What Foods To Be Wary Of

Caveat Emptor (Buyer Beware)

You have just dined and however scrupulously the slaughterhouse is concealed in the graceful distance of miles, there is complicity.

Ralph Waldo Emerson

Joan, age 34

I eat when I am stressed out and have a huge problem that needs solving and I just don't know what to do. Ninety percent of the time the issue is financial stress, wondering how will I pay for this or that, like braces for my daughter. I sit down and pig out on fast foods—junk, cheeseburgers, pizza, French fries, fats—until my stomach actually hurts. I'm in pain from being overfull, but I can't stop. I feel horrible; I think that I need to stop. I get no relief from the problem—in fact, now I have double stress, the original stress, plus the stress from overeating. I feel guilty and say, "it will never happen again" and try not to think about it further, but it happens a few times every month.

My objective in this chapter is *not* to dictate authoritative advice to not eat *this* or not eat *that* particular item of food. My intent is to simply point out that there are many unhealthy foods ready for the taking, and that we would be best served by not overdoing it with the consumption of such foods that can promote obesity and an unhealthy existence. To put it tersely: as <u>heal</u>thy food can heal, so can un<u>heal</u>thy food un-<u>heal</u>. The eating goal for mankind should be to nourish man kindly—to become healthier, eat healthier foods. Healthy eating is the simplest and least expensive means of maintaining our good health and well being.

On a practical basis, it is extremely difficult, if not impossible, to maintain an ideal diet all of the time. My intention is to increase awareness of foods to which the adage "everything in moderation" should be applied with particular diligence.

> We need to preserve the right to opt out or our grand-children will have no choice but to eat amalgamated, irradi-ated, genetically-prostituted, bar-coded, adulterated fecal spam from the central processing conglomerate.
>
> Joel Salatin (from Michael Pollen's *The Omnivore's Dilemma*)

Regarding what to eat to maintain good health, the celebrated author Michael Pollen famously stated: *Eat food, not too much, mostly plants.* I borrow his maxim and reverse it in an effort to sum-marize what to eat to promote poor health: *Eat imitation food, eat a lot of it, mostly animal-based.* And there we have the *Western diet*—processed foods, lots of meats, refined carbohydrates, fats and sugar—the eating style that has contributed to two-thirds of us Amer-icans being overweight or obese. The *Western* diet is largely respon-sible for the diseases of Western civilization, namely hypertension, diabetes, cardiovascular disease and some cancers.

Processed Food: *Nutritional Fraud*

Much of what we eat is not actually food, but *enhanced food-like matter*, highly processed and laden with additives, preservatives, and loaded with fat, sugar, salt and other chemicals (most of which are unknown, unpronounceable, unrecognizable, un-food-like concoc-tions)—engineered in a science lab. Processed foods can be defined in several different ways. The Industrial Food Complex defines processed foods as: *attractive and marketable food products produced by the transformation of raw ingredients using harvested or slaugh-tered components.* A more realistic definition is: *real food that has been altered in order to lower its production cost, lengthen its shelf life, make it look more appealing and make us want to eat more of it, resulting in a reduction of nutritional content and an increase in chemicals, dyes, preservatives and toxins.* Another definition might be: *reconstituted, unhealthy, mystery muck* or, alternatively, *faux foods* or *ersatz eats.*

Minimizing one's exposure to processed foods, as difficult as that might be, is a noble idea in terms of avoiding being overweight or obese and maintaining good health. Examples of processed foods are: Pop Tarts, Hostess Twinkies, Spam, hot dogs, Doritos...the list is virtually endless. Processed foods can be as detrimental to our health as tobacco has been proven to be. Years ago, smoking was an excusable habit simply because we did not know any better. Please note my words—there will come a time when processed foods will be understood to be as harmful as tobacco is—it may take some time until this concept gains traction, but I predict it will ultimately come to fruition.

WHO KNEW? When I lived in California for a year during my fellowship training at UCLA, I often started my day with one hour of aerobics at the painful hour of 6AM at the Sports Connection Fitness Center. After an invigorating shower, I would commute into Westwood, and before heading to the office I would stop at McDonald's for a breakfast consisting of black coffee and a raspberry Danish pastry. I truly thought I was being "healthy," drinking coffee without dairy products or sugar, and avoiding bacon, sausage and cheese. Little did I know that the pastry was full of enriched wheat flour, partially hydrogenated vegetable oils, trans fats and high fructose corn syrup—a vicious combination of coronary artery clogging, unhealthy calorie-rich and nutrient-poor processed glop. Had I known, there would have been no way that I would have started my day with that kind of breakfast. How ironic that I put so much effort into staying fit by arising early and really 'bringing it' at the fitness center only to undermine my efforts by eating such an unhealthy meal!

The term *processed* is a derivative of the word *procession*. A procession is a movement that occurs in an orderly fashion, for example, a parade. The procession that results in processed food on our plates involves the *farmer*, the *processor*, the *baker*, the *distributor*, the *retailer*, and ultimately us, the *consumer*. For example, wheat is grown and harvested by the farmer and the process of *threshing* separates the wheat kernels from the chaff (husks of the wheat grains). The process of *milling* enables the wheat kernel components to be separated such that the bran and germ are removed, leaving the pure, silky, highly refined powder that we know as wheat flour. This wheat flour is then used as one of the many unhealthy components of processed foods, for example—a Twinkie. After the Twinkie is configured, baked, sealed in plastic wrap and boxed, the distributor trucks and ships the product to our local supermarket retailer where we can purchase it. So what starts out as a healthy and natural grain, after much processing, ends up as unhealthy junk food. The final product bears little relationship to the original farmed product. The bottom line is that the more that is done to our food, the more it gets depleted of its nutritional value.

Remember the game called "telephone" we used to play when we were kids? A bunch of us would sit in a circle and the first person would whisper a few sentences into the ear of the person sitting next to him or her. That person would repeat it to the next person, and so on around the circle. The last person would announce the message they heard. The message that the final person announced was virtually always very different and distorted from the original message, usually in a very funny way. My point is that the processing of food is not unlike this game in that the final product bears little, if any, relationship to the original, with each step in the production process resulting in increasing adulteration.

As much as I am denigrating processed foods, it is important to understand that not all processed foods are bad and that food processing is a necessity. We all cannot be farmers and grow a variety of vegetables and fruits and raise cattle and other livestock. We must rely upon intermediaries to transform a raw product such as wheat grain into an edible form. However, the desirable goal is to eat a healthy, nutritious, robust, wholesome processed product, for example, 100% whole grain wheat bread vs. the infamous un-wholesome Twinkie. Obviously, the closer any food item resembles its original and natural form, the healthier it is, but many original forms do need to be processed to some extent to make the food *available* to us. In general, real food comes from the earth and not the laboratory, and the less processing the better. The corollary of this is that the more processed and highly altered the food is, the less nutritious—and oftentimes more deleterious—it becomes.

Processed foods are generally unhealthy and nutritionally void and have an abundance of sugar, salt, fat, additives, preservatives, flavor enhancers, chemicals, and dyes. Some processed foods are filled with mystery components. Often, to make up for loss of nutrients during processing, synthetic vitamins and minerals are added. Consuming a diet high in processed foods can contribute to diabetes, obesity, hypertension, cardiovascular disease and cancer.

As I sit here re-reading and editing this manuscript, I am in a lovely hotel in New Orleans, sipping on a cup of coffee as my wife and daughters are sound asleep. I made the coffee in my room and picked up a package of "creamer" to look at the ingredient list, which read as follows: corn syrup solids, partially hydrogenated soybean oil, sodium caseinate, dipotassium phosphate, mono and diglycerides, sodium silicoaluminate, sodium tripolyphosphate, diacetyl tartaric acid esters of mono and diglycerides, artificial flavor, beta carotene, riboflavin, titanium dioxide (artificial color).

Reminds me of high school chemistry lab . . . .Thank you, no . . . . I'll take my coffee black!

The *"Killer"* Triad

The "killer" triad of processing is *enriched wheat flour, high fructose corn syrup* and *partially hydrogenated vegetable oils*. These products are ubiquitous in many processed foods, junk foods, and fast foods. The only way we would ever know that we were consuming these products is by developing the habit of reading the nutritional label on the back of every package or can. Simply by reading every food label carefully, we can obtain significant insights into the component ingredients as well as their nutritional values or lack thereof. Labels now exist on nearly all supermarket purchases, are easier than ever to comprehend, and will give us some basic facts regarding the nutritional value of food items before we decide to buy them, prepare them, or consume them. The ingredients are listed in descending order of predominance. If we read the ingredient list of a Twinkie, we will see in addition to the aforementioned killer trio—that is, enriched wheat flour, high fructose corn syrup and partially hydrogenated vegetable oils—the presence of *beef fat, preservatives, artificial colors* and *artificial flavors*. It was news to me that a Twinkie was an animal product!

Food should be thought of in many ways as a drug, and we are on a *need-to-know basis* about the component ingredients. We should be as mindful regarding food consumption as we are about medicine consumption. The following questions should come to mind before putting food into our mouths just as they should before taking a medication: What are the reasons for taking it? What is in it? What are the side effects? Is it safe? We would never think of taking a medication that was dangerous to our health, unless the benefits outweighed the adverse effects, yet many of us consume foods that are unequivocally detrimental to our health.

Modern food production involves a wide range of chemicals, many of the processed foods that we eat being engineered in a science laboratory. Food scientists are responsible for these laboratory experiments, and we do not want ourselves or our families to be the subjects of these experiments! So, before we purchase a package of food, we need to carefully scrutinize the list of ingredients. Processed food products typically have a long list of ingredients that are often unfamiliar or unpronounceable. If the list is lengthy, it is probably best to leave the package on the shelf. Likewise, if the list has unpronounceable chemicals—a chemist's list of ingredients added by food scientists—this is probably an item that we do not want to consume. Remember, real food comes from Mother Earth and not the chemistry lab. In general, too, packages that make health claims—often evidence of processed food within—should be abstained from. Real food does not need to make health claims—*res ipsa loquitur* (the thing speaks for itself).

Now a few words on the processing of grains—specifically wheat, since these *amber waves of grain* are staples of the American diet; however, this same general discussion is germane vis-à-vis other grains including rice, corn, rye, oats, barley, etc. Highly efficient, modern technology milling enables the wheat kernel to be separated into the following three components: the *bran*, the outer covering of the wheat kernel; the *germ*, the embryo or sprouting section; and the *endosperm*, the source of the white flour that contains starch and protein. White flour has the bran and germ removed, resulting in a pure, highly refined powder as opposed to whole wheat flour that contains the bran and germ. By removing the fiber-rich bran and germ, the resulting product has a longer shelf life and makes for lighter and fluffier breads, as opposed to the darker, coarser, heavier breads made from the whole grain wheat.

The removed bran and germ—the wholesome and healthy components of the wheat kernel—are often used to produce animal and poultry feed. So the farm animals are fed the wholesome, slow-digesting grain components and the humans eat the refined and unhealthy component. Go figure! In fact, the nutritionally depleted and deficient processed white flour needs to be fortified with vitamins and minerals to replace those that were lost in the refining process, hence the term "enriched" wheat flour.

So what is the problem with *enriched wheat flour*, the first ingredient in the vicious triad? Simply stated, wheat grain that is hulled and strip-mined of the bran and germ results in a pulverized, superfine, silky white powder. This highly refined substance is very similar in appearance to cocaine or heroin. This pre-chewed-pre-digested-melts-in-your-mouth-adult-baby-food equivalent is absorbed quickly and is rapidly transformed into glucose; it is not too dissimilar from getting an injection of intravenous glucose into one's bloodstream. This *quick fix* of sugar is not particularly filling because of the absence of fiber—it is a short-lived satisfaction that begs for more consumption, establishing a vicious cycle. The result is a push in the direction of weight gain, insulin-resistance, obesity, diabetes and heart disease. Furthermore, this refined product does not induce the *thermic effect* that many more substantive foods do, in which the body's metabolism increases because of the energy expenditure it takes to digest a wholesome, fiber-rich product.

In contrast to the refined, enriched wheat flour product, *whole wheat flour* is made by grinding the *whole* grain of the wheat kernel. "Whole" refers to all grain components used—bran, germ, and endosperm. Whole wheat flour is brown in color and textured, as opposed to the silky-white enriched wheat product. Whole wheat is very nutritious because the bran and germ components contain abundant fiber, protein, calcium, iron and other minerals. Because of the fiber, glucose transformation and absorption occur in a slow, gradual and well-regulated fashion. Whole wheat is filling, satisfying, and substantive and literally *sticks to your ribs*. Whole wheat adds heaviness to breads or to whatever recipe it is used for and requires more flour to obtain the same volume of bread as white flour. Whole wheat has a shorter shelf life than white flour because of its higher oil content—the source of the oil being the wheat bran, and the oil being a healthy one. Whole wheat flour is also more expensive than white flour. It is easy to understand why the Industrial Food Complex is enamored with enriched wheat flour!

Let us now get to the subject of the second of the killer triad—*high fructose corn syrup (HFCS)*. HFCS is a sugar substitute that is derived from corn via a complex enzymatic process. Without going into excessive detail, corn is milled to produce cornstarch, a powdery derivative. The cornstarch is processed into corn syrup, which contains the glucose. Glucose is converted to fructose by using a process developed in the 1970's by food scientists in Japan. Glucose is then added back in differing percentages to the fructose to achieve the desired sweetness. A 55% fructose HFCS is used to sweeten soft drinks and a 42% fructose HFCS is used in baked goods. HFCS is ubiquitous in processed foods and beverages with the typical American consuming approximately 70 lbs of HFCS on an annual basis!

Why does the Industrial Food Complex adore HFCS? It is less costly than sugar because of corn subsidies and sugar tariffs. It is easy to transport as the viscous syrup lends itself to transportation in a huge storage vat within a truck, similar to how gasoline is transported. Fructose is the sweetest of all naturally-occurring carbohydrates and does not crystallize or turn grainy when cold, as sugar can do in cold drinks such as iced tea. Because HFCS is highly soluble, its use makes for softer products and its ability to retain moisture allows for moister and better textured baked goods. Finally, it acts as a preservative to help prevent freezer burn as well as maintain the freshness and extend the shelf life of processed foods. While HFCS may help preserve processed foods, it does not help preserve us!

So why do our bodies *not* like HFCS? Fructose is different from glucose in that it is metabolized differently. Whereas every cell in our bodies can metabolize glucose, only the liver can metabolize fructose. Fructose does not stimulate insulin release as does glucose, nor does it stimulate *leptin* secretion, which functions as our satiety hormone. Fructose more readily than glucose replenishes liver glycogen, and once the liver is replete with glycogen, triglycerides (fats) are made and stored. Thus, HFCS ingestion can readily lead to obesity, elevated cholesterol and hypertension. The bottom line is that excessive HFCS ingestion pushes our metabolism towards fat production . . . and it doesn't take eating that much processed food to cross the excessive HFCS threshold! (It should be noted that table sugar, consisting of 99.9% sucrose—a glucose-fructose mix—is biochemically similar to HFCS, although the jury is still out on whether the two are metabolized differently; however, sugar remains a refined and processed product that should also be used in moderation.)

Fructose is the predominant sugar in many fruits, hence the name *fructose*. The difference between this sugar contained within a piece of fruit as opposed to that within a bottle of cola is that fruit fructose is natural (not created in a chemistry lab) and the amount is significantly less than the load contained within the soft drink. Additionally, the fruit fructose is accompanied by a substantial amount of fiber, anti-oxidants, and other phyto-nutrients, all health-promoting ingredients lacking in the cola.

The third component of the deadly triad is *partially hydrogenated vegetable oils*. First, a few words on fats, to put this third component in proper perspective. Fats as macronutrients have been given a bad rap, and as much as any of us do not want to have excessive body fat, nonetheless, fats are rather important to us. They are a very efficient means of energy storage, fat having more than twice the calories per unit weight than carbohydrates or proteins. They cushion our internal organs, insulate our bodies and are an important component of cell membranes and brain cells. Dietary fats can be animal or plant based. Fats consist of chains of fatty acids and the fats circulating in our blood and stored in our fat cells are known as triglycerides. Oils are simply liquid fats.

Fats are classified in terms of their *saturation* with hydrogen. In general, the more saturated the fat is, the more unhealthy it is because it is the saturated fats that are the ones that cake and clog our arteries. *Saturated fats* are solid or semi-solid at room temperature, for example, animal fat, butter and tropical oils. *Unsaturated fats* can be either mono-unsaturated or poly-unsaturated. *Mono-unsaturated fats* include peanuts, cashews, walnuts, pistachios, macadamia nuts, canola oil, olive oil and avocado. *Poly-unsaturated fats* include safflower, sunflower, sesame, corn, flaxseed, soybean and fish oils. Mono-unsaturated fats and poly-unsaturated fats are known as "good" fats because they can actually lower cholesterol levels and diminish our risk for cardiovascular disease, as opposed to the saturated fats, aka "bad" fats, that elevate cholesterol and promote cardiovascular disease.

Tropical oils include palm, palm kernel and coconut oil. Palm oil was introduced as a plantation crop and is inexpensive, produced year round, and prolongs the shelf life of products it is used in. Even though they originate from plants, tropical oils are more similar to beef tallow than vegetable oil and are more saturated than pig fat. They are perhaps better described as *axle grease, tree lard* and *cow fat disguised as vegetable oil*. So, even though they are not animal fats, palm oil and other tropical oils such as coconut oil and palm kernel oil are so saturated that they behave like animal fats. Clearly, they are too saturated for our good health and are better suited for use in sun block and skin moisturizing lotions...which they are! Beware of consuming any chemicals that are also products in moisturizers and cosmetics!

Now, with that background in mind, let us get to the matter of *partially hydrogenated vegetable oils*. They are made via a process in which relatively healthy oil—a natural unsaturated fat—is pumped up with hydrogen, thus chemically converted into a fat that is solid at room temperature. And so are born products including margarine and vegetable shortening. What starts as a soybean, for example, is processed into soy oil, which is then converted into the vegetable shortening that we might use to make cake frosting.

Trans fats are by-products of the hydrogenation process. They are not fully saturated, but are mono- or poly-unsaturated *unhealthy* fats. Suffice it to say that trans fats are solid at our body temperatures and are difficult to metabolize. They are unhealthy because they increase our bad cholesterol, decrease our good cholesterol, and promote arterial deposition and plaque formation that leads to cardiovascular disease. Fortunately, there has been widespread dissemination of information on the unhealthy nature of trans fats and many restaurants and school systems nationwide have already eliminated foods containing trans fats from their menus.

So why is the big food industry smitten with partially hydrogenated vegetable oils? Simply because of their superior baking properties and prolonged shelf life since they are less prone to turning rancid, decreasing refrigeration requirements. They may prolong the shelf life of food, but they do not prolong our shelf life! They are used ubiquitously in processed foods, particularly baked goods such as cookies and cakes. Why does our body *not* like partially hydrogenated vegetable oils? In addition to the trans fats created as a by-product of the chemical process, the hydrogenation increases the saturation of a healthy vegetable oil; it is the saturated fats that are solid at room temperature and that have a propensity to clog our arteries, promoting a myriad of health problems. Clogged arteries are never good—compromised blood flow to our organs will not allow delivery of oxygen and vital nutrients and can engender heart attacks, strokes, peripheral vascular disease, etc.

Scary Stuff

Aside from the vicious triad and tropical oils and trans fats, what other food items or ingredients are not healthy for us?

Chemical preservatives are added to many foods to keep them fresh, extend their shelf life, and slow the process of spoiling. These preservatives are abundant in packaged and processed foods. Remember, real food comes from the earth and not the laboratory and does not have or need chemical preservatives added. In my opinion, it is best to try to avoid chemical additives including preservatives, and try to eat wholesome, fresh, natural and robust foods—avoiding packaged, processed, preservative-laden items whenever possible.

There are three types of chemical preservatives: *antimicrobials, antioxidants, and enzyme-targeters*. Antimicrobials include *calcium proprionate, monocalcium phosphate, benzoates, sorbates, nitrates* and *nitrites*. Nitrites and nitrates are used to color, flavor, and preserve meat products including bacon, ham, hot dogs, luncheon meats, etc. Their benefit is that they help prevent botulism in these processed meats, but the problem is that they react with amino acids to form nitrosamines, which are considered to be carcinogenic. Antioxidant preservatives, such as *butylated hydroxyanisole (BHA), butylated hydroxytoluene (BHT)* and *propyl gallate* slow the oxidation of fatty acids that can cause rancidity, and there is similar concern that they may be carcinogenic. A third group of preservatives targets enzymes in the food itself that continue to be active—the enzyme phenolase, for example, functions as soon as an apple or potato is cut, causing the exposed surface to brown. *Citric acid* and *ascorbic acid* inhibit phenolase and are not harmful to our health. *EDTA (ethylenediamine tetraacetic acid)* is another example of a preservative in this category. *Sulfur dioxide* and related *sulfites* work as preservatives by all three of the above-mentioned mechanisms.

Artificial colors and *dyes* have been linked to cancer in laboratory animals. I'm not sure how this translates to humans, but nonetheless, all things being equal, if we have an opportunity to avoiding eating foods containing an artificial color or dye, we should act upon that opportunity. Artificial colors and dyes are best suited on palettes, canvasses, and in clothing, but not in our bodies. *Natural*, i.e., occurring in nature, will always trump artificial in my way of thinking. In fact, the word *artificial* when it comes to food—in any dimension—does not make me sanguine. This goes for *artificial flavors, artificial sweeteners* and *artificial fats* like Olestra. Fake foods are fine for displays and for children playing "kitchen" in the basement, but when it comes to eating, we want to nourish our bodies with the real thing.

The consumption of a healthy, balanced and wholesome diet, free from *hormones, antibiotics, pesticides,* and *bacteria* is a reasonable expectation. Healthy, balanced and wholesome is not that difficult of a proposition if you put your mind to it. However, food sans hormones, antibiotics and pesticides is not a diet that is easily achievable, nor inexpensive, although it is possible by eating organically-raised produce and meats.

In the livestock industry, *hormones* are used to accelerate weight gain and reduce the time to slaughter, as well as to increase milk production in dairy cows—resulting in increased profits for the meat and dairy industries. *Recombinant bovine growth hormone* is sometimes used to boost the milk production of dairy cows. A variety of steroid hormones are used to promote livestock growth, including the following: *estradiol, progesterone, testosterone, zeranol, trenbolone acetate,* and *melengestrol acetate.* I am concerned about the ramifications of these hormones with respect to our health, particularly insofar as synthetic steroid hormones have been found to pose a cancer risk. Studies to date have not demonstrated any deleterious effects on our health from the small amount of residual hormones in meat or dairy products, but if truth be told, I would rather not be ingesting any amount of synthetic hormones in the food that I eat.

Antibiotics are mixed in animal feed by agribusiness companies in an effort to keep their livestock healthy by compensating for the typical unsanitary, crowded, and inhumane feedlot conditions and to promote faster growth and hasten the animals' time to market. This is in extreme contradistinction to animals raised under humane circumstances with adequate living space and appropriate foods. The very same classes of antibiotics that are used in human beings are used in the animal factories. In fact, approximately 70% of all antibiotics used in the USA are used in the factory feedlot industry! This has definitely contributed to the emergence of bacteria that are resistant to antibiotics—a very real problem that physicians confront every day in our medical practices. Close to 100,000 Americans die annually from hospital-acquired infections, 70% of which are caused by bacteria that are resistant to at least one potent antibiotic. Because of increasing prevalence of the antibiotic resistance problem in humans, many scientific organizations are urging the powers that be to eradicate the non-therapeutic use of antibiotics in livestock.

Pesticides are typically used on produce including fruits and vegetables in order to protect them from the ravages of their predators. The problem is that a certain amount of these toxic chemicals remains on the produce. The government sets and regulates the maximal amount of pesticide residue remaining on fruits and vegetables at a level known as the "tolerance" level. The highest levels of pesticide residues are on the following produce items: peaches, strawberries, apples, sweet peppers, celery, nectarines, cherries, pears, imported grapes, spinach, lettuce, carrots, frozen winter squash and potatoes. It is controversial about the harm that these substances may do to us, but all things being equal, I sure don't want to be ingesting pesticides.

Yikes, but many of us eat lots and lots of fruits and vegetables! So what can we do? We can thoroughly wash produce before consumption. Peeling will help, although at the cost of the loss of lots of nutrients in the skin. Unfortunately, many of these pesticides are absorbed directly into the fruits and vegetables and thus cannot be washed or peeled off. Alternatively, we can buy organic produce in which chemical pesticides have not been used, probably a very good idea for those fruits and vegetables that have very high levels of pesticide residue. The down side is that organic produce is very costly.

Fecal bacterial contamination of our foods is an increasingly prevalent problem and one that has received a significant amount of publicity—to wit, numerous disturbing reports on E. Coli 0157:H7 contamination of hamburger meat resulting in recalls. The astonishing and frightening lead articles on the front page of the October and December 2009 *New York Times* by investigative reporter Michael Moss cannot help but make us question whether we ever really want to eat another hamburger again. He won the Pulitzer Prize for his article entitled, "The Burger That Shattered Her Life," describing the horrible E. Coli illness linked to the consumption of Cargill ground beef by a young woman.

Fecal bacterial contamination of livestock is viewed by the government and meat suppliers as acceptable and a given at certain levels. However, even a small amount of contamination—a collateral effect of what animals are fed and how they are raised—can make us very ill, or in some instances, even cause death.

If we buy ground beef off the shelves of a supermarket, what we actually get is an amalgam of various grades of meat from different parts of cows and different slaughterhouses, both nationally and internationally. One hamburger may represent a composite of up to 1000 cows! The more cows and the more slaughterhouses involved in the ground beef, the greater the risk of fecal contamination. There exists strong potential for bacterial E. Coli contamination during every single step of beef processing. And so it would seem that the only way for us to get a hamburger that originates from one cow and dramatically reduce our potential for E. Coli exposure is by purchasing a cut of beef and having our butcher grind it up for us—I'm told brisket makes for an amazing burger.

A company called Beef Products, Inc., came up with the "clever" concept of using the lowliest waste products of the beef carcass— fatty slaughterhouse trimmings with no functional value, typically used for pet food and cooking oil—as a means of keeping the cost of hamburger meat as low as possible. This company conceived the novel idea of treating the fatty trimmings with *ammonia* to kill the bacterial contaminants, particularly E. Coli and Salmonella, prevalent because of the low grade and quality of beef remnants used. The ammonia works no differently than it does for household cleaning, the alkalinity of the ammonia causing bacterial death. Unfortunately, the ammonia has not proven to be a failsafe measure of sterilization, and there have been numerous instances of bacterial-contaminated beef . . . plus, who wants to be consuming ammonia, a product that truly belongs on our kitchen floors!

Beef Products' meats are widely used in fast food restaurants, including McDonalds and Burger King, as well as in the ground beef sold in supermarkets and used in the federal school lunch program. School lunch officials allow hamburgers served in schools to contain 15% of the product, which serves to bring the price down. Some customers have complained about the ammonia-like taste and the pungent odor of their beef. Ammonia is not listed as an ingredient on the label, but is referred to by the moniker "processing agent." A former USDA microbiologist, G. Zirnstein, commented that the beef product is a "pink slime that I do not consider to be ground beef, and I consider allowing it in ground beef to be a form of fraudulent labeling."

E. Coli 0157:H7—a type of bacteria that is responsible for hemorrhagic colitis and a myriad of other health problems, even including death—is often contracted by the consumption of contaminated beef, although it can also occur by eating spinach and apple juice contaminated from the fecal run-off from farms that raise cattle. E. Coli 0157:H7 is a product of two factors—the *corn* that the Industrial Food Complex feeds cattle and the feedlot where the cattle are raised.

Cows are hard-wired to eat *grass*, but since corn is cheap, convenient and every kernel contains a big dollop of starch (corn has been bred to contain more carbohydrates and less protein), it will make for bigger and fatter cattle. We all know how too many "carbs" make us humans fat, and the same is true for other mammals. These literally *obese* cattle will get to slaughter faster and yield beef that is well-marbled with saturated fat that commands a higher ranking on the USDA beef hierarchy and translates into more dollars and profits for the industry. The beef from grass-fed cattle is different than that from corn-fed cattle, essentially being less marbled with saturated fats, healthier, and less likely to be contaminated with E. Coli and other such bacteria.

Since the digestive system of ruminants like cattle did not evolve for the digestion of large quantities of corn, their consumption of corn—as opposed to grass, the staple of a ruminant mammal's diet—changes the bacterial content of the cow's stomach, allowing for the emergence of E. Coli. Under circumstances of a grass diet, stomach acidity results in the death of most of the bacteria within a cow's stomach.

Cattle raised on grass on real ranches via traditional pasture farming lead a much different life from cattle raised on feedlots, which are the large industrial factories where most cattle are raised in over-crowded and contaminated environments. These animal factories are known as CAFOs (Confined Animal Feeding Operations). It is to some extent similar to the difference between living leisurely in an affluent suburb on a large piece of land, versus a crowded, infested, and dangerous inner city environment. Cattle raised in feedlots stand in very filthy and over-populated conditions, ankle-deep in manure, with their hides caked with excrement, overfed with starch-rich corn and further fattened by their limited availability to move around. The use of antibiotics in the feed is, in fact, an attempt to neutralize some of this fecal contamination.

The problem occurs in the slaughterhouse where the more manure on the animal, the greater the risk of fecal contamination upon processing the animal. Cattle often arrive with smears of feedlot feces on their hides and when the knife is brought to the flesh, the meat can get exposed to bacterial contaminants that are present in the cow feces. Ground beef, in particular, lends itself to contamination because its constituent parts are often the lower quality parts of the cow that are more likely to have fecal contact. There is additional risk of E. Coli contamination at the gutting station, where the intestinal tract—where E. coli resides—is separated from the rest of the animal.

So what to do? There are a number of possible solutions. We can cook our hamburgers so that they are so well done—ala hockey pucks—that bacteria don't have a fighting chance. We can forego meat and become vegetarians or vegans. We could select *certified organically-raised beef* that has far less chance of contamination. In the ideal world, certified organic beef is derived from a ranch that maintains a record of breeding history and veterinary care rendered to its cattle. The cattle do not receive hormones or antibiotics, are fed organic grains and grasses, have unrestricted outdoor access, and are treated in a humane fashion. Alternatively, we can purchase meats from local farmers or at farmers markets. Or we can go to a reliable butcher and pick out a nice cut of meat and have him grind it in front of us. Or we can try the DIY (Do It Yourself) approach and raise a few head of cattle in our backyards (try getting a town or city permit for this one!).

Nullius in verba (take nobody's word for it): I hate to throw a fly in the ointment, but is organic really *organic*, or is it mere semantics? Are organic livestock pasture-based? Prior to June 2010, at which time more stringent rules went into effect, the requirement for organic *dairy* producers was the following: *organically-raised livestock had to have access to pasture.* Theoretically, this might mean that a farmer permitted his cattle pasture time for 10 minutes each day—a mere romp in the field allowing for the label "organic." This was a loophole allowing some dairies to feed their animals almost exclusively a diet of grain feeds. The new regulations state that cows must now graze on pasture for a major portion of the grazing season—a minimum of 120 days mandated by law—and must get at least 30% of their food from pasture during the grazing period. These new rules also apply to beef cattle, with the exception that the 30% requirement is suspended during the 4-month period when the animals are fattened prior to slaughter. Ahhh . . . yet another disturbing loophole in the quest for truly grass-fed cows!

In New York City there are now several *Shake Shack* restaurants where, in contradistinction to your typical fast food restaurant, you can get what seems to be as close to a healthy burger as you possibly can. Right off their menu is the following: *whole-muscle, no-trimmings, fresh-ground, antibiotic-and-hormone-free, source-verified-to-ranch-of-birth, choice-or-higher-grade Black Angus beef.* Sounds like a great option when that carnivorous craving strikes!

And now a little aside on American-grown poultry exported to Russia and Europe, according to a *New York Times* report by Michael Schwirtz in January 2010. Russia's view is that American poultry is fatty, tasteless and raised on chemicals. From Russia's perspective, the critical issue is that American companies use *chlorine* to disinfect the poultry after slaughter. Russian health officials feel that the chlorine method is unsafe and outlawed it in 2008, as had the European Union previously. The Russian government imposed a ban on the importation of American chicken, purportedly because US companies have been remiss in adhering to Russia's new food safety regulations. Prime Minister Putin stated that the USA was not ready to observe Russian poultry standards. *Yikes, so we use chlorine to disinfect our chickens, just as we do to decontaminate our pools and our standards are not good enough for Europe and Russia!*

Another healthy alternative chosen by many is to buy *kosher* meats. Kosher foods—prepared in accordance with Jewish dietary laws and requiring certification—have really come into their own in this era of food fears engendered by numerous reports of food contamination, food allergies, and the dubious provenance of many ingredients. Forty percent of the food items sold at supermarkets now bear the kosher imprint and only fifteen percent of those who buy kosher do so for religious reasons. The vast majority of those who buy kosher, including an increasing number of non-Jewish people, do so because of the perceived high quality, purity of ingredients and healthiness, thought of in a similar vein as *local* and *organic* foods. Is kosher food actually any healthier or safer than non-kosher food? The honest answer is that we just don't know.

The Food Chain

It is the sun that is the source for our energy from food as all nutritional energy originates as *solar energy*. Plants, including the oceanic biomass, use solar energy to fuse carbon dioxide and water to create glucose, which is the most basic food substance of plants and animals. This process is called *photosynthesis*. As a byproduct of this process, oxygen is released into the environment. Pretty amazing if you think about it—carbon dioxide plus some water and some sunshine and plant cells magically make glucose, releasing oxygen—completely clean and efficient. At night, after the sun has set, the reverse process occurs whereby glucose combines with oxygen to break down into carbon dioxide and water, releasing energy in the process. This process is called *respiration*. Also pretty amazing—literally a plant is able to store the energy of sunshine and release it for energy use at night!

Within the framework of the food chain, animals consume the plants, and humans consume the animals and the plants—thus, nutritional solar energy is responsible for the energy that empowers our lives. Plants are the fundamental intermediary agents for the transfer of this solar energy to humans.

We are what we eat—the very foods that we eat literally become part of our body's structure in addition to providing us with a source of energy. The cells that compose the tissues and organs of our bodies are in a dynamic state and are constantly sloughing, regenerating and renewing themselves—the foods that we ingest are the very ingredients in their recipe for cell repair.

We are what we eat eats—if what we eat eats something not so good, then we eat something not so good. For example, the nutritional content of that salmon that we ate for dinner reflects what the salmon ate or did not eat. If it was a wild salmon from Alaska, its diet was very much different from the factory-raised variety from a salmon farm. Farmed salmon are fed fishmeal, fish oil and grains—these are typically treated with antibiotics, parasiticides and vaccines because of crowded pens making the fish more susceptible to infections such as sea lice. The farmed salmon may harbor up to ten times as many pesticides, PCBs (Polychlorinated Biphenyls), dioxins and mercury toxins as Pacific wild salmon that subsist on a diet of smaller fish and plankton. So, whatever diet our salmon consumed is going to be reflected in what shows up on our plates...and consequently, what winds up in our bodies.

We are what we eat eats eats and so on—this is getting a bit confusing now, but this is nothing other than the *food chain*. For example, wild salmon from Alaska consume fish known as wild krill, and what krill eats will be reflected in the nutritional content of the wild salmon on our dinner plates. We as humans sit on the very top of the food chain, and it is very important that we know precisely what is in our food since toxins get more concentrated with each rise in level of the food chain. One reason that a vegetarian diet is healthier than an animal-based diet is simply because a vegetarian diet is lower on the food chain—thus it contains less environmental toxins since such toxins tend to get increasingly concentrated the higher up the food chain we go.

Questionable Cuisine

Now, a few words on some specific "pet peeve" foods: *doughnuts*—nutrient-empty, fat-laden sugar balls—the only healthy part of which is the hole in the center (in other words, no doughnut at all!). *Hot dogs* sure do taste great on a nice, soft bun with mustard slathered all over, but in my opinion, they are just not worth it. They go down easy, but they are a bitter pill to swallow! Why? Simply because they are nothing other than *undesirable fatty animal parts ground into a homogeneous composite and stuffed into a synthetic casing, drowned in preservatives—toxic waste in a tube*, if you will. The same may be said of many other cured luncheon-type meats—salami, bologna, pepperoni and other "mystery" meats. I always wonder about anything that is *ground up and reconstituted*—clearly, if someone is grinding up bits and pieces and then putting them back together into one combined unit, that someone is likely trying to hide the presence of some very undesirable components! What is it exactly they are hiding in there? If truth be told, I don't really care to find out! There are whole foods—*integral foods* if you will, for example, apples—in which what you see is what you get—and then there are foods that consist of a mélange of ingredients mixed together and prepared. I propose that if we could see the precise ingredients that go into making many recipes—particularly processed packaged foods—we would be somewhat more reluctant to eat them. The final product simply hides all the component ingredients. When it comes to hot dogs and similar type foods, I would be so bold as to state that were it possible to see the component ingredients laid out in front of us, our relationship with this kind of food would be brought to an abrupt halt!

Fast foods, with occasional exception, are the quintessential unhealthy dietary development of modern times. To me, they can be thought of as *greasy, fat-laden, calorie-dense, low-fiber, over-salted, queasy-engendering, bad aftertaste-in-your-mouth junk*. On occasion, fast food is unavoidable, so if we have no other options (such as when we are traveling), we can opt for the salads or the broiled, not fried, meal alternatives. That being said, fast food chains of recent have been making a real effort to serve healthier and reduced-calorie alternatives, and this concept seems to be gaining traction. Subway, Dunkin' Donuts, Taco Bell, McDonald's, among other fast food franchises, have made claims that they offer sandwiches that are low in calories and fat. It is noteworthy that they are all *loaded* with sodium—far in excess of what would be considered healthy—and an additional caveat is that if high-fat condiments are used, they will mitigate the lower fat and calorie benefits.

Salt is one mineral that should be consumed in moderation. Excessive salt intake can contribute to high blood pressure, weight gain, fluid retention, heart failure, etc. The daily recommended amount of sodium is only about 1500 milligrams (mg), which is less than one teaspoon (one teaspoon of salt contains about 2300 mg). Three-fourths of the salt we consume is from processed foods. Beware the sodium content of prepared and processed foods, especially canned soups, deli items, cottage cheese, salad dressings, and breads. By reading labels, we can easily become aware of the salt content of the foods that we are eating. Unfortunately, restaurant foods are loaded with salt and there is no way of knowing their salt content. The January 2010 *New England Journal of Medicine* reported that by consuming even a relatively smaller amount of sodium, we can reduce the number of cases of heart disease and stroke as much as can weight loss, cholesterol lowering, and giving up cigarette smoking!

What to drink? We are now drinking more calories than ever before in the form of *sweetened drinks*—sodas, teas, punches, etc. The problem is that these empty calories are the equivalent of *liquid candy* and do not provide satiety, but do supply us with a large bolus of calories that clearly has contributed to the obesity epidemic. The lion's share of the sweetener used in these products is high fructose corn syrup, obviously an unhealthy choice.

How about good old water? As reported in *The New York Times* in December 2009 by Charles Duhigg, over the course of the last five years, more than 20% of the water treatment systems in the USA have violated major provisions of the Safe Drinking Water Act, the law that requires communities to deliver safe tap water to local residents. Chemicals including arsenic, radioactive uranium, the dry cleaning solvent tetrachloroethylene and dangerous microorganisms such as bacteria, viruses and parasites have been identified in our drinking water. These contaminants have been linked to numerous instances of illness and some of the chemical contaminants are carcinogenic. In fact, the water supply of the cozy suburban town that I reside in is contaminated with arsenic! The Environmental Protection Agency has been remiss in their responsibility of enforcing the Safe Drinking Water Act by fining or sanctioning only a small fraction of the municipal water systems in violation of the law.

Bottled water has certainly become increasing popular with the average per capita annual consumption in the USA being about 30 gallons. Most of us are completely unaware that up to 50% of bottled waters come from municipal sources—aka tap water! The Food and Drug Administration (FDA) regulates bottled water as a food under the Food, Drug and Cosmetic Act and is responsible for ensuring that bottled water is safe and truthfully labeled, whereas the Environmental Protection Agency (EPA) regulates tap water. The FDA establishes allowable levels for chemical, physical, microbial and radiological contaminants. There are microbiological standards that set allowable bacterial levels; physical standards that set allowable levels for turbidity, color and odor; and radiological standards that set levels for radium-226 and radium-228 activity, alpha-particle activity, beta particle and photon radioactivity, and uranium. The standard of quality also includes allowable levels for more than 70 different chemical contaminants. The FDA has generally adopted the EPA's standards for maximum levels for contaminants in tap water as the same allowable for bottled water and the EPA's maximum residual disinfectant levels for disinfectants and disinfection byproducts. Just recently, the FDA mandated that bottled water manufacturers test source water for total bacteria and require a determination as to whether any of the microorganisms are E. coli, indicative of fecal contamination. Of note is a recently released report by the Environmental Working Group—a non-profit agency dedicated to consumer protection—entitled "2011 Bottled Water Score Card." It raises considerable questions as to the source, purification/treatment methods, and contaminant levels of 173 popular bottled water brands. Disturbingly, most of them received poor to failing grades regarding the above-mentioned concerns.

So what to drink? It remains a confusing, disconcerting conundrum as to whether bottled water overseen by the FDA is any better and safer than the tap water regulated by the EPA. We have to drink. So our choices are tap, bottled, boiled, distilled, filtered, or water that has been subjected to some sort of purification process such as reverse osmosis, ultraviolet light exposure or ozonation. Knowing what we know about water contamination, it is definitely prudent to use some form of purification system if it is tap water that we choose to drink. If bottled water is our choice, perhaps paying heed to the Environmental Working Group's safety rating list is advisable.

Is water contamination any great surprise to us? Collectively, human imprudence and greed have been rather unkind to Mother Earth. *What goes around, comes around*, i.e., *cosmic karma*—for years we have polluted the air, water and soil of the earth and are now paying dearly for it—we have been wanton in our actions and our folly is coming back to haunt us. Our power plants, vehicles, refineries and industrial facilities have spewed horrific volumes of exhaust gases, smoke and by-products of coal combustion into our air. We have dumped billions of tons of industrial effluents, mining and agricultural wastes and raw sewage into our rivers and oceans. We have polluted our soils with chemicals from herbicides and pesticides and have overfilled landfills with garbage and toxic materials. There are well over 1000 Superfund toxic waste cleanup sites in the USA! Our civilization has stripped the earth, mined it, burned it, consumed its natural resources, deforested it, emitted into it . . . basically, we have raped and pillaged and destroyed much of it. We have paved over large swathes of the earth in an effort to urbanize and industrialize the land...and are now at the point where there is much less of anything clean and natural left.

This life of ours is not a board game: Just by virtue of our being able to transport, shift, and compartmentalize our waste into discrete dumpsites, basically a lose-lose strategy of taking hazardous matter from point A to point B, does not liberate us from their ill—likely deadly—effects. In essence, our now "Going Green" may be too late since we "Went Red" a long, unfortunate time ago. What happens to the inhabitants of the planet is a microcosm of what happens to Mother Earth, since we—and almost all that we eat—breathe the air, drink the water, and eat the food grown in the soil.

We are *entitled* to know the *provenance* of our food and drink— its origin and source serving as a guide to its authenticity and quality. However, the Industrial Food Complex has deliberately obscured this information from us. We literally do not have a clue as to where our food originates from, what exactly it is that we are consuming or what it is doing to our bodies. Farming and ranching are now big businesses using an assembly line-mass production-factory modus operandi that maximizes profits by keeping manufacturing as well as consumer prices affordable. Mergers and consolidation in the food and agribusiness sectors have resulted in the survival of only a small number of giant multinational corporations that wield tremendous power with respect to our food supply. Monsanto dominates the domestic seed industry with control of more than 90% of soybeans and 80% of corn grown. Tyson, Cargill, Swift and National Beef Packing Company dominate the beef packing industry with over 80% market share and Smithfield, Tyson, Swift and Cargill govern the pork packing industry with almost 70% market share. As a result of this corporate agribusiness mentality, food has become much more dangerous in ways that are being purposely hidden from us. There is a tremendous need for transparency regarding the entire process from which a raw material is transformed into a product that we purchase in the supermarket.

In summary, the consumption of healthy foods untainted by chemical additives or contaminants is nothing short of a challenging, if not a daunting, proposition. It is easy enough to be nutritionally conscientious and carefully read labels in an effort to be food savvy and avoid many of the chemicals that have been added to our foods by processing. Even if we heed Michael Pollen's famous words—*Eat food; Not too much; Mostly plants*—with the utmost of solicitude and diligence, the challenge remains. Our cognitive brainpower and five senses can inform us to some degree if a food is healthy, fresh and edible, but are not sophisticated enough to discern chemical tainting. Obviously, the closer that any particular food resembles its original and natural state, the healthier it usually is—with the corollary being that the less a food resembles its native state, the unhealthier it usually is. It is a given that with highly processed foods such as—*you fill in the blank (take pepperoni for example)*—the final product is many iterations removed from nature, the provenance of the components is truly unknown, and there are so many opportunities for chemical and biological mischief to occur. However, even with, for example, an apple—a natural fruit that processing has left largely unperturbed—we are incapable of detecting whether there are agrochemical pollutants or contaminated residues remaining on the fruit that are potentially deleterious to our health. The soil that the apple tree grows in may largely be a mystery, with the potential for contamination. Based upon current reports, even the water that we use to water the apple tree and that we use to cleanse the apple is possibly unhealthy for us! What to do then? We can only do the best that we can do in an effort to remain diligent to minimize our exposure to the barrage of biochemical insults that we are subjected to daily.

Is Processed Food Really Any Different From Tobacco?

Both tobacco and processed foods share many qualities. Whether it is nicotine or a formulated glob of processed sugar, fat, and salt—cravings, dependency and addictive and habit-forming behavior can result—perpetuating the desire for more and more of the product. There are 46 million smokers in the USA and surveys show that 70% desire to quit, 40% per year try to quit, and 2.5% actually succeed.

Clearly, tobacco is very bad for our health, with 400,000 Americans succumbing to smoking-related diseases each year. At one time we simply were ignorant about the ill effects of tobacco—now we are educated and informed—so lack of knowledge is no longer a valid excuse for smoking. Nowadays, those who choose to smoke make a conscious choice of *ignoring* available information about the harms of tobacco as opposed to the *ignorance* of years ago.

It is my contention that the consumption of unhealthy processed foods is no less toxic and harmful to our health than tobacco is. Of course, it is difficult to quantify—I do not know the relative harm of a Hostess Twinkie as compared to a few cigarettes—but with the knowledge that we now have, it is crystal clear that both habits are pernicious to our good health.

It took many years to come to an understanding of the incredible health risks due to tobacco and how far tobacco companies went to wantonly inflict these hazards upon us. In response to a 1952 *Reader's Digest* article entitled "Cancer by the Carton" that revealed the dangers of smoking, big tobacco started mass-marketing filtered cigarettes and low-tar formulations that promised a "healthier" smoking experience. In 1964, it was concluded that cigarette smoking was causally related to lung cancer in men on the basis of carcinogens including cadmium, DDT, and arsenic. In 1965, Congress passed the Federal Cigarette Labeling and Advertising Act mandating the Surgeon General's warnings on all cigarette packages. In 1971, all broadcast advertising for tobacco was banned and in 1990 smoking was banned on all interstate buses and all domestic airline flights lasting six hours or less.

In 2006, a federal judge named Gladys Kessler ordered strict new limitations on tobacco marketing, punishing the cigarette manufacturing companies for their disingenuous behavior and forcing them to stop labeling cigarettes with deceptive descriptors including "low tar," "light," or "natural." The tobacco industry was demonstrated to have "marketed their lethal product with zeal, with deception, with a single-minded focus on their financial success and without regard for the human tragedy or social costs that success exacted." Judge Kessler concluded that "cigarette makers profit from selling a highly addictive product that causes diseases leading to a staggering number of deaths per year, an immeasurable amount of human suffering and economic loss, and a profound burden on our national health care system."

The Industrial Food Complex—a small group of multi-national corporations that are responsible for most of our foods—are similar to big tobacco in their size, power and resources, commanding the whole food system from seed to supermarket. It is becoming increasingly evident that the Industrial Food Complex controls the farming and meat industries, which are no longer so much farms and ranches as they are manufacturing plants. Much of our food comes from huge assembly line factories where, to put it bluntly, both animals and workers are treated very poorly without the respect, dignity and common decency that they are owed. The IFC conducts their business with opaqueness and does not care for us to know the truth about what we are consuming and the means by which we have come to consume it, very similar to the attitude of Big Tobacco towards cigarettes. The goal of the IFC is to make produce or livestock bigger, fatter, cheaper and brought to market faster—all with the intent of increasing their bottom line—with significant collateral costs to us in terms of damage to our ecosystem and health-related problems, including bacterial contamination of our food and the increasing prevalence of obesity, diabetes, cardiovascular diseases and some cancers.

The IFC shares with the cigarette manufacturing companies a propensity for dishonest and deceptive behaviors. Many processed products that are perilous to our health are neatly packaged and boxed with marketing claims that can be described as sly-manipulative-spun-hyped subterfuge. There is often a sleight of hand applied to the number or the size of servings delineated on the package, with a realistic-sized serving being much larger and higher in calories than stated. Another example is the ingredient listing on the package, ingredients being listed in descending order of predominance. Many breakfast cereals are predominantly sugar, but if sugar were listed as the primary ingredient, many consumers would choose to leave the product on the supermarket shelf. So the IFC's magic trick of deception is to use multiple sweeteners and list them separately—sugar, brown sugar, high fructose corn syrup, corn sweetener, molasses, and honey are the typical menu of sweeteners. By using more than one sweetener, they drop down on the order list and are seemingly less predominant components. Like Big Tobacco, Big Food also uses many deceptive descriptors including: "fortified," "lite," "multigrain," "all natural" and "organic"—they sound great for our health, but really are just words without substance. The term "all natural" resonates nicely but is meaningless—many things are all natural including E. coli O157:H7 and malignant melanoma. "Multigrain" conjures up images of a mélange of farm-fresh healthy grains, but in reality translates to made from more than one grain, all of which may be highly processed. "Organic" is a powerful "halo" term that evokes thoughts of food grown without the use of chemical fertilizers, growth hormones, antibiotics or pesticides. However, understand, for example, that when I walk my English Springer Spaniel to do his "business," he leaves a large, steaming pile of *organic* material on the ground!

It is now common knowledge that tobacco is deleterious to our health and we are slowly coming to an understanding that processed foods are equally harmful. However, it took years for public attitudes to change and for a grass roots understanding and acceptance of tobacco as a malignant addiction to solidify—to wit, when the Surgeon General's warning first proclaimed that smoking was bad for your health in 1964, 42% of the adult population smoked, and now in 2011, about 20% does so. Ultimately, government and anti-tobacco forces assailed smoking from a number of different angles—prohibiting smoking in public venues and restaurants, levying higher taxes, banning commercials and mandating warning labels on packs—cumulatively acting to gradually erode the smoking base. In a similar vein, it will likely take some time for the public to recognize and accept that processed foods are harmful to our health and existence. Mark my words—there will come a day when processed foods will be understood to be as harmful as tobacco—it may take years for this transformation to occur, but it will ultimately come to fruition when the coalition of government and community advocacy groups as well as grass roots forces join ranks to change the food culture of our society.

In 2003, the Big Tobacco Company formerly known as *Philip Morris* changed its name to *Altria* in order to rid itself of the "scarlet letter" tainting its public image that was so tarnished because of its cigarette business. Same company—new name—how calculating and disingenuous can you get? Will the Big Food Industry companies be following suit? What game playing and charades!

The tobacco industry has been shown to be irresponsible and just recently—finally—the government rose to the occasion with sweeping new legislation to control it. Half a century after the Surgeon General first warned about the deleterious health effects of tobacco, and despite the opposition of the omnipotent tobacco lobby, 2009 ushered in the passage of landmark new laws that gave the FDA comprehensive powers to oversee and regulate tobacco. The government first required warning labels to be printed on cigarette packages in 1965 and updated them in 1984. Now, regulators will control the amount of addictive nicotine in each cigarette and how cigarettes are packaged, marketed and promoted. Larger and more graphic warnings of the perils of smoking will be on every pack of cigarettes. Now banned are fruit-flavored cigarettes and using, for advertising purposes, cartoon characters that are attractive to youngsters (like Joe Camel)—restrictions aimed at preventing children from picking up this horrendous habit.

I foresee the day when—like the tobacco industry—the Industrial Food Complex will be censured and intensely regulated for zealous and deceptive marketing practices and for their primary focus on their own prosperity with patent disregard to the human tragedy and social costs resultant from that prosperity. We are in dire need of legislation capable of preventing children from starting down the misdirected path that can lead to obesity, diabetes, cardiovascular disease and premature death. Hopefully happening sooner rather than later, these regulations and restrictions directed at the Industrial Food Complex will force transparency; big and obvious warning labels instead of enticing catchwords; control of the amount of high fructose corn syrup, partially hydrogenated vegetable oils, enriched wheat flour, and the many other harmful component ingredients; and regulation of packaging, marketing and promotion. I anxiously await the time when the public understands that highly processed foods—in similar fashion to tobacco—can be extremely addicting and contribute insidiously to diseases leading to an astonishing number of deaths, human suffering, economic loss and a significant burden on our health care system.

I look forward to the day when unhealthy foods bear the Surgeon General's warning. There are currently four such warning on cigarettes that are rotated from pack to pack: *Smoking Causes Lung Cancer, Heart Disease, Emphysema and May Complicate Pregnancy; Quitting Smoking Now Greatly Reduces Serious Risks to Your Health; Smoking By Pregnant Women May Result in Fetal Injury, Premature Birth, and Low Birth Weight; Cigarette Smoke Contains Carbon Monoxide.* Perhaps the food warning label will read something like: *Consumption of Processed Foods May Contribute to Obesity, Diabetes, Cardiovascular Disease, Cancer And Death*; or alternatively, *Quitting Consumption of Processed Foods Now Greatly Reduces Serious Risks to Your Health.* In my opinion, that day cannot arrive soon enough.

CHAPTER 4

Psychological Perspectives

The Mind Vis-à-Vis Eating— Battling Raw Emotions with Food

Carly, age 40

When I am stressed or have things on my mind or I am really tired, I eat sweets, like cakes and cookies. I don't even give it any thought. I feel bad after and think about eating better or exercising, but I don't act on these thoughts. I really don't care so much about how I look, but I care about my health because I need to be around to take care of my babies.

The Mind-Body Connection

Although it is convenient to think of our minds and bodies as separate and discrete entities, our emotional and cognitive abilities do not exist independently of our flesh and physical beings. Our minds and bodies are very much commingled, and our mind-body connection is profound. Our bodies house our minds, and our minds control our bodies, but our minds are made of matter just as our bodies are, and our bodies have a vast array of neural networks running through them that essentially are peripheral extensions of our minds. When our minds are unhealthy, often our bodies become unhealthy, and vice-versa. Optimal human functioning and performance requires a coordinated, synergic and harmonious relationship between our minds and bodies. An understanding of our mind-body relationship is fundamental in the effort to conquer eating issues.

The following are a few examples of my own mind-body connection in action:

When I was in third grade, my mother visited my elementary school classroom, observing the class being taught. Prior to leaving, she walked to my desk and, in front of the entire class, gave me a big smooch on the cheek. My face was crimson in color for hours.

I was recently operated on for a ventral hernia—not really a major ordeal, but when positioned on the operating room table I stared nervously at the headlights above, and my pulse bounding with anxiety and fear that was beyond my control. I was so tense that I felt my body trembling and my heart pounding in my chest like a bird fluttering its wings in a cage!

After ten hours or so of seeing patients, I often find myself exhausted and very stressed. My usual routine is that upon arrival home, I change into workout clothes and head downstairs to the basement to exercise. After a good workout followed by a nice, hot shower, I emerge—physically and emotionally invigorated, my stress released and fatigue having gone by the wayside—to join my family for dinner with a refreshed outlook and a heady sense of well being.

The above show how our minds can affect our bodies—blushing from embarrassment and the classic physiological stress response; and how the body can affect the mind—physical exercise transforming an emotional state. The essence of the mind-body connection is that our thoughts, feelings and emotions can affect our body chemistries and cause a physical response, and conversely, our physical actions, like exercise or laughter, can influence our brain chemistries and affect our thoughts, feelings and emotions. We can utilize our understanding of the mind-body connection to help re-educate and ultimately re-program our neural pathways to promote a change to a more mindful and healthier eating style.

Consciousness

At one time or another, all of us find ourselves gliding through life in a *mindless* and *semi-conscious* state—existing in a bit of a fog, not really paying careful attention to what is going on *around* us or *within* us. Mindlessness is not dissimilar to the state of mind associated with *highway hypnosis*—we stare out blankly ahead in an altered state of awareness, unfocused on the road, the car seemingly moving on autopilot mode with little to no conscious recollection of having traveled many miles. It is certainly never a good thing to bring a mindless state to driving an automobile, playing a sport, or for that matter, to any aspect of life. Being focused, in touch, present in the moment, having purpose and bringing our best state of consciousness to any endeavor is to our advantage in terms of performance and profiting from our experience.

I picked up a book this morning and "read" a couple of paragraphs and soon came to the realization that I had not comprehended one word. My eyes had swept appropriately across the page and I clearly visualized every word, but the sentences could have been written in Greek as to my understanding of them. My mind was simply elsewhere. This is an example of mindlessness—mindless reading. At least I was attentive to the fact that I was being inattentive. I restarted the ignition to my mind and reread the paragraphs; now fully mentally engaged, I easily comprehended the written words.

Consciousness can be defined as the state of being awake and aware not only of our external environment and surroundings, but also our internal environment—our mind's awareness of *itself*. There exists a huge spectrum between the extremes of full *consciousness* and the vegetative state marked by *unconsciousness*. All of us are familiar with being in an intermediate state between these two extremes, typified by the dream-like states of falling asleep and awakening. Altered states of consciousness go far beyond sleep time and can occur during awake life, as exemplified by the aforementioned example of highway hypnosis. Alcohol, other medications, and a variety of emotions can engender an altered level and quality of consciousness. In other words, emotional engagement can affect our state of consciousness and mindfulness and our state of consciousness can profoundly affect our behaviors, including eating. Anything that is capable of interfering with pure and undiluted consciousness— that which messes with our heads—can confound our relationship with food. The emotional "baggage" that we carry around and which preoccupies us uses up some of our mind's resources, allowing fewer resources for general mindfulness. When this combination of compromised mindfulness is coupled with a strong urge to pacify an emotion, mindless eating is often precipitated, and foods containing sugars, fats, salts, etc., are often the *seeming* solution.

David Brooks, op-ed columnist for *The New York Times*, at a recent interview provided some valuable insights into consciousness versus subconsciousness. We are capable of processing our environment on a conscious or a subconscious basis. Data and information is processed largely without our conscious awareness of the acquisition, with a miniscule amount that we are consciously aware of. His metaphor for conscious/subconscious is a "general" and "scouts," respectively—our conscious is a general in charge, looking down from above, whereas our subconscious are the scouts out in the environment who send emotional signals to the general. The yarn of our experiences and beliefs informs our subconscious.

How often I have read a book or sat through a lecture at the conclusion of which I questioned what I had learned. In actuality, I had learned quite a bit, but was simply unaware of the process of acquisition. When laser-focused mindfulness is brought to any endeavor, the mind becomes so thoroughly engaged that we lose touch with our environment and the passage of time. This can happen when reading a great novel, watching a gripping movie or participating in a meaningful conversation—we are "transported" beyond our immediate environment.

Mindfulness vs. Mindlessness

Mindfulness denotes a calm awareness of our feelings, the content of our consciousness, and consciousness itself. Mindfulness implies not just being there, but being fully present—*bringing it*—to any activity. Mindfulness is a critical factor in the path to enlightenment with respect to any undertaking. In my favorite tennis instructional book entitled *Winning Ugly*, Brad Gilbert, Andre Agassi's tennis coach for many years, famously summarized the essence of mindfulness in the following paraphrased words: "The mind is a terrible thing to waste; most recreational players are mentally lazy, long on running and short on thinking, and it is imperative when playing tennis to know who is doing what to whom."

Mindfulness is not an easy state to achieve; in fact, it is a *difficult* state to achieve and even harder to maintain. Mindfulness requires effort and concentration. It takes much less effort to exist in a mindless daze than with mindful focus. Mindfulness takes work and needs to be cultivated. Mindfulness requires *mindfulness*. Analogously to how we use our eyes to peer into our eyes, and how our hearts beat to provide blood to our organs and so to the heart itself— similarly our minds' mind must be engaged to cultivate mindfulness—the mind must be able to attend to itself.

Mindfulness when applied to eating behavior refers to reflective, aware, attentive, in touch and tuned-in eating. Mindful eating is done with a sense of purpose as opposed to reflexive eating that seems not to involve our higher brain centers. Mindful eating implies knowledge of salutary benefits of healthy eating and the detrimental effects of unhealthy eating. It also involves *passionate* eating—taking the time to see, smell, hear, touch and taste food—eating slowly and deliberately to savor the experience and appreciate the moment, as opposed to *perfunctory* eating. Mindfulness will result in eating in a healthier, better and smarter way and can help eliminate obsessive thoughts about foods, control cravings of specific foods and avoid overeating.

Mindlessness, when applied to eating behavior, refers to when we eat in a manner that is reflexive, inattentive and tuned out to the various dimensions of eating, i.e., mindlessly chomping away or eating like a ravenous dog. Mindlessness also implies a lack of knowledge of the salutary benefits of healthy eating and the detrimental effects of unhealthy eating. Mindless eating is a style of eating in which we do not allow ourselves to see, smell, hear, touch, and taste food—eating rapidly and thoughtlessly with no savoring of the experience nor appreciation of the moment. When we eat mindlessly, we are likely to eat much more than we desire to consume, since we are just not being attentive.

Alan, age 47

Eating is my best friend—it makes me feel good. Filling the void in my stomach once filled the void in my life. I used to eat massively, for example, four bagels every day for breakfast six days a week. I was a Wall Street trader and had to put up with great amounts of stress, but every emotion imaginable—happiness, sadness, ecstasy, depression—would trigger my eating. I used to wait for my wife to go to sleep so that I could go down to the kitchen and eat unobserved. I would eat any food. My eating is a psychological disease. I lost 140 lbs with the help of Overeaters Anonymous. My glucose went from 400 to 100, but my diabetic neuropathy persists.

Promiscuous Eating

When I use the term *promiscuous eating,* I am not referring to smearing chocolate erotically on the body of your lover! The appellation *promiscuous* eating is defined as the wanton, reckless, indiscriminate, casual and intemperate consumption of foods without regard to the potential consequences of this indiscretion. This is as opposed to *mindful* eating in which thought is given to our eating, with every effort to make the wisest and most prudent food choices—foods that will promote our health rather than promote disease; foods that are in their closest state to nature as possible; foods without dangerous additives, chemicals, dyes, hormones, antibiotics, pesticides, preservatives and processing.

A meaningful and healthy interpersonal human relationship most often implies a sustained, sound and steady commitment with another compatible and quality human being. In similar fashion, a meaningful and healthy relationship with what we eat implies a long-term commitment to quality foods and eating for the right reasons, in the right place, at the right time, in the right manner. A healthy relationship with food will not cause us to feel guilt or regret or disgust the next morning as promiscuous eating might.

If we are consistently and knowingly making poor food choices that are deleterious to our health, it can be considered to be promiscuous eating. If food is being consumed for purposes other than satisfying genuine hunger, it might be deemed to be promiscuous eating. That being said, the concept of eating as a form of *entertainment* and the anticipation and enjoyment of a good meal is not in any way to be construed as promiscuous. However, if we are watching television or reading on the couch while mindlessly wolfing down food, it can be judged to be promiscuous eating. If we ingest two peanut butter and jelly sandwiches at 3AM when we have a bout of insomnia, it can be deemed to be promiscuous eating. If we shovel a half-gallon container of double-fudge ice cream right out of the carton or devour an entire bag of sour cream and onion potato chips, it can be regarded as promiscuous eating. An extreme example of promiscuous eating is when we scarf food while we are sitting on the toilet bowl, doing our "business"—no, I kid you not, this happens!

Matt, age 54

I eat when I'm pissed—for example, when my wife rags on me. I will eat a box of Devil dogs—10 or so—it makes me feel better.

In the process of promiscuous eating we consume *stealth calories*—calories that we sneak into ourselves and, with rare exception, are not usually enjoyed in the process, leaving us bloated, fatter and often feeling angry and guilty. Mindless caloric consumption often does not permit appreciation of what we are eating or attention to the quantity of intake. When the mind is turned off, it opens up a huge potential for eating problems.

The short-term consequences of promiscuous eating can be guilt, distress, unhappiness and feelings of repugnance towards ourselves, aside from the physical feelings of bloating and sometimes queasiness. The long-term consequences of promiscuous eating can be obesity, diabetes, hypertension, cardiovascular disease, cancer and premature death.

The most radical and extreme form of promiscuous eating is *bulimia*, a psychological eating disorder characterized by binge eating followed by inappropriate methods of compensation for the bingeing including vomiting; fasting; laxative, enema or diuretic use; or compulsive exercising. Binge eating involves the extraordinarily excessive, out-of-control consumption of calories, not driven by hunger, but in response to psycho-emotional matters such as stress, anxiety, depression or self-esteem issues. The individual who suffers with bulimia will often experience disgust and self-loathing after the binge. Unfortunately, the bingeing/purging cycle often becomes an obsessive behavioral pattern. *Binge eating disorder* is defined as at least one binge weekly for at least three months, with the consumption of platefuls of food, rapidly and to the point of discomfort, accompanied by severe guilt and plunges in mood. This is a serious psychological disorder that requires professional help, without which there can be dire medical consequences.

Most of us, after overeating for any reason, will feel some variable degree of guilt, regret, disgust or remorse. Simply stated, we feel badly about the consumption of unnecessary calories. The vast majority of us will give it some thought and resolve not to engage in this type of eating behavior again, and some of us will compensate through more disciplined restraint and augmented physical activity for the few days following such an over-indulgence. The problem is, like New Year's resolutions, few of us are capable of staying true to our vows and declarations, and in a matter of days we are back to business as usual. This disconnection between our thoughts and our actions seems to be a most universal, human phenomenon. Driven by nature itself, we are programmed and hard-wired to enjoy eating—it is one of our biological imperatives. Fighting nature is a very challenging proposition. In the battle of nature versus the will of mankind, man will rarely be the victor, and this is likely one of the reasons why weight loss and weight maintenance are such difficult and challenging propositions. Only a very finely honed and determined will, contingent upon uber-mindfulness, can possibly prevail.

On so many levels, it makes a great deal of sense to avoid promiscuous eating behaviors. It is fundamentally important to try to recognize precisely what it is that triggers such eating patterns. Triggers may be stress bringing on the need for comfort, the desire for stimulation driven by boredom, or the longing for sedation spurred by anxiety or depression. Additionally, lack of sleep, positive moods such as happiness and fulfillment, and for that matter, any state of altered consciousness can engender promiscuous eating. The loss of inhibition resulting from the consumption of alcoholic beverages or other drugs can also lead to eating with abandon.

Insofar as eating is a highly sensual and almost sexual activity that brings a great deal of enjoyment to many of us, it is easily liable to addictive tendencies and promiscuous behaviors. The solution to avoiding promiscuous eating is the cultivation of a strong sense of mindfulness about every aspect of eating. The first step is recognition and admission that an eating issue exists and identification of triggers. Of critical importance in preventing such dysfunctional eating habits is an awareness of *what, why, when, where, how* and *how much* we are eating. Eating the right foods in the right quantity for the right reasons will help to keep us on track. Being nutritionally conscientious, food savvy and consuming healthy and wholesome foods in a slow, deliberate and mindful manner, thus allowing for the savoring of the experience, is most desirable. Full-throttle mindfulness is the key to maximizing our ability to maintain a healthy relationship with food and avoiding obesity and all of the potential harmful medical consequences that can arise from mindless and promiscuous eating patterns.

Kim, age 30

I am an anxiety eater. I am a single mom with three young kids, a homeowner with lots of bills and an ex-spouse who I am angry at and who does not provide child support. During my 45-minute drive home, I stop at Dunkin' Donuts for a coffee and a bagel or at a gas station for chips. I eat them in the car while driving. Half of me says to eat, the other half, not to eat. I get no pleasure out of this and get angry with myself after. It is worse when I am stressed and tired. I have gained so much weight that the only clothes I wear at home are loose jogging attire.

Psychological Perspectives and Eating

Food can be considered or interpreted from different perspectives and vantage points. Let us take, for example, a piece of fresh fruit. On a *visceral* and *instinctual* level, it can be thought of as a bright, colorful and fragrant enticement that is available and begging for consumption. On the other hand, from a *cognitive* and *mindful* perspective, it can be thought of as a wholesome and natural food that will not only be pleasing to the taste and other senses, but will also provide us with energy, nutrients and antioxidants that will promote our health and well being and furnish us with nourishment and satiety.

When a reptile with its primitive reptilian brain stares its prey in the face, it is unlikely that it is considering its meal on any level beyond a "gut" level. We humans, however, with our highly evolved central nervous system, are indeed capable of a higher order consideration of our "prey." And therein lies the problem—our highly evolved-cognitive-rational-mindful-enlightened capabilities are a double-edge sword—we have the capacity for higher order thinking and experiencing richly textured emotions, but these very same emotions can interfere with our sophisticated mindfulness and drive dysfunctional, mindless and promiscuous eating behaviors. Furthermore, these emotions and feelings can cause us to seek any solution that might subdue and neutralize them, and it is often our "prey" that can provide this. The saving grace is that our mindfulness, encompassing full consciousness and self-awareness, can inform us of exactly what we are doing and why we are doing it and the means of rectifying the problem.

Eating is simply so much more than *eating*. For most of us, the consumption of food is a highly enjoyable and sensual activity, piquing all of our senses. It is an important undertaking in terms of social bonding and fostering relationships with family, friends and business associates. Eating serves a major role in our celebrations, recreation and rewards. Because eating is pleasurable and because numerous emotional factors can influence our eating—stress, anxiety, happiness, depression, mood swings, etc.—the potential for overindulgence exists, leading to obesity and a myriad of other health problems.

Each of us, including people of *any* weight or body mass index, has a relationship with food—sometimes it is healthy, sometimes unhealthy, but it is typically unique and complex for each of us. If we are concerned about our weight, it becomes of fundamental importance to learn and understand how we relate to food and whether or not the relationship is working. If the relationship is not functioning satisfactorily, in order to effect a change in our weight, we will need to modify and amend our relationship with the food that we eat.

Elana, age 52

I am a type A plus, tightly controlled person who runs, spins and does Pilates seven days a week. I eat a really healthy diet, being basically a vegetarian, but I also eat seafood. I usually have a small breakfast and lunch, so when I get home I am starved and somewhat stressed and tired, having dealt with people all day long. I am conditioned to eat whatever is available, but since I eat very healthy foods, I usually have things like veggies, edamame, whole wheat products, vegan snacks, fruits, and sunflower seeds. I might eat an entire head of lettuce, so much volume to the point where I have abdominal pains. I feel that I have an insatiable appetite and eat way too much and it makes me feel guilty afterwards. Once I start snacking, it's just difficult to stop. It's really not about being hungry—it's more a part of my "winding down" process—my routine—just me and my salad to help me chill and mellow out. This is very personal and I do this only when alone, not when I'm with friends or dating. When I change my routine and go out for dinner, when I get home, even though I am not hungry and it's late, I am conditioned to eat something, usually rice cakes—because I haven't had that "personal time." When really upset, I eat nothing; when going through a divorce, I lost 10 lbs. Wine causes me to lose control.

The aforementioned vignette is an excellent example of the very unique relationship that each of us has with the food that we eat. It also demonstrates that emotional eating patterns occur even in extremely fit and athletic individuals who are very attentive to their diet. Emotion-driven eating can occur regardless of body size, gender, age, race, etc.

The Vicious Cycle: *Prompt-Impulse-Act-Compensation*

Although a wide range of emotions can trigger eating, let us use stress as an example, since it is probably the most universal emotion that drives eating. (However, we could use any other emotion including boredom, anxiety, depression, happiness, or any altered state of consciousness.) Stress or anxiety can act as a *prompt* (something that induces us to action) to drive an *impulse* (an impelling force) to eat. If the impulse is carried to fruition, the *act* (behavior) of eating occurs. If the act results in *compensation* (alleviation of the stress or anxiety), the act of eating is reinforced and sets up a *behavioral pattern* (a repetitive and predictable set of responses) for the future. This ultimately becomes a vicious cycle that converts the act of eating in response to certain emotional states of mind into an ingrained pattern. This cycle is predicated on the profound relationship between our mind and body.

The aforementioned cycle has a neuro-biological basis. Humans have pleasure "pathways" located in an area of the brain known as the *amygdala*, a temporal lobe structure that is the part of the limbic system involved in memory and emotional processing. Through the processes of *neuroplasticity* and *adaptation*—the ability of the brain's neurons to undergo anatomical changes and reorganization of their networks with new neural connections generated in response to new situations or environmental changes—learned pleasurable behaviors actually modify the electrical hard-wiring of the brain, which is dynamic and constantly subject to change. As a behavioral pattern becomes firmly established, neural pathways are modified in such a way (synaptic "sculpting") as to facilitate the repeated behavior. Thus is explained on a biological basis how a behavior becomes ingrained. The good news is that just as behaviors can be learned, they can also be unlearned (synaptic "pruning") because of the plasticity of the system.

For example, let's use the two glazed doughnuts that I consumed every evening at 10PM as a freshman at Middlebury College. An enterprising student made the doughnut rounds in the dormitory and I found them irresistible, a soothing tonic to the stress and anxiety brought upon by the first semester in college and a demanding pre-medical curriculum. My nocturnal habit of regularly consuming these gooey, sticky, sugary treats contributed towards my gaining 20 lbs or so by winter break.

The *prompt* was the stress, the *impulse* to eat led to the *act* of the doughnut consumption and the *compensation* was the stress relief derived. Fortunately, I was ultimately able to give up this seemingly innocent but pernicious *behavioral pattern* that was not doing me nor my waistline any good at all. I came up with the following thought process: *doughnuts have more than 500 calories; they make me feel disgusting; my weight gain, which I find abhorrent, is in a large part on the basis of these late-at-night unnecessary calories; my tight pants repulse me; I went jogging in Florida with my brother over winter break and could not keep up with him because I was so out of shape.* This is opposed to the following lines of thought that goaded me to consumption: *doughnuts taste great and are something to look forward to after the tedium of studying for hours on end; they soothe, calm and sedate me; I owe myself this reward because of my hard work; I do not wish to deprive myself.*

So, the concept of *mindfulness* came into play and disrupted what had become an ingrained pattern of behavior. Essentially, in psycho-speak, mindfulness functioned to un-condition the link between the *compensation* and the *prompt*, to disrupt the cycle. Mindfulness and cognitive focus—on many levels—can help us to deal with situations similar to the one that I experienced as a college freshman. Both the internal prompt of stress/anxiety and the external prompt of seeing the tray of doughnuts being paraded around the dormitory helped drive my behavioral pattern. Mindfulness is a useful tool when applied to figuring out what drives the internal prompts and how to deal with them in an appropriate and healthy manner.

In my example, the stress and anxiety from the change of life of moving away from home and starting college, as well as the intensity of studying, etc., drove the desire for "compensation." As we all have to adapt in response to changes in our environment, so would I adjust to this new life, and I would need to learn to deal with my emotions in a healthier and more appropriate fashion. I substituted swimming for the doughnut habit, a much more suitable activity! Once again, it came down to the mindfulness of swapping an alternative behavior—exercise—equally effective as a doughnut or two in terms of dealing with stress and anxiety, believe it or not. An additional effective tool is that in knowing how we may succumb to our weaknesses, we can limit our exposure to such external prompts, which in my case was by purposely avoiding the doughnut vendor.

Whether the prompt is "managed" by comfort foods or exercise, the same "cocktail" of internal chemicals, including endorphins, is released into our bloodstreams, resulting in compensatory relief of the altered emotional state. We are *all* stressed to some extent, and one thing for sure is that stress is unlikely to disappear any time soon. If it is not one source of stress, it will be another. So when the root cause is not necessarily remediable, the next best bet is to deal with it in a healthy way—healthy in terms of psychological, emotional and physical health. So why not seek relief with the more appropriate and healthy means? I could also have had the mindfulness to trade the doughnut consumption for a healthy replacement food item such as an apple. As hard as it might be to believe this, nowadays I actually prefer apples to doughnuts and cannot remember the last time I indulged in *nutrient-empty, fat-laden sugar balls* (alright, I do confess to recently having had a beignet at Café du Monde in New Orleans, but it was a very special occasion!).

Mindfulness again: Thinking about my college doughnut indulgence, I realized that by giving in to my impulses, I merely received the benefits of a short-term and temporary reward that did not truly address the problem at hand. In psychological terms, this enabled and facilitated a vicious cycle and a dysfunctional habit and thus the creation of a secondary problem . . . .now I faced stress over school as well as stress over my unseemly weight gain. By actively not indulging my impulses, I managed to weaken the behavioral pattern that had been established, helping to break the cycle. I did lose those 20 lbs, but by no means was that an easy feat.

Psychology 101 As It Relates To Eating

There are a number of psychologists whose works are relevant to our behaviors with respect to food and eating. I have selected a few—Freud, Pavlov, Skinner, Csiksczentmihalyi, as well as the French author, Proust. My intent is to summarize their seminal contributions and discuss how viewing our eating behaviors through the prisms of their perspectives and philosophies can provide us with insight and understanding of not only why we eat for emotional reasons, but also to help us eliminate our inappropriate eating behaviors.

Why bother learning the philosophy of the aforementioned psychologists and authors? Many intelligent people I have spoken with tell me that they don't really care about the psychological underpinnings of their eating behaviors, only about how they can achieve weight loss and keep it off. So how can this knowledge improve our ability to get to a healthy weight and stay there? The answer is because when we eat for the wrong reasons and emotions drive dysfunctional eating patterns, we must be cognizant of our behaviors and make every effort to understand them in order to change them. Freud's divisions of the psyche, Pavlov's classical conditioning, Skinner's operant conditioning, Csiksczentmihalyi's concept of flow, and Proust's "Madeleine" each offer a unique framework to comprehend the basis of human behaviors, including eating. Even more importantly, these formative contributions offer insights into how to manage dysfunctional eating behaviors in order to achieve the endpoint of a healthier relationship with food, healthier eating patterns and a healthier weight.

Freud

The model of the human psyche established by Sigmund Freud divides our psyche into the *ego, id* and *super-ego.*

Our *ego* acts in accordance with the *reality principle.* The domain of the ego is conscious awareness, reason and common sense. Our ego is responsible for the delicate balance between primitive drives and reality, essentially mediating between the two poles of the id and super-ego. Our ego can be thought of as the *adult* within.

Our *id* operates in accordance with the *pleasure principle.* The domain of the id is instinctual impulses, drives and passions that demand immediate satisfaction. Our id can be thought of as the *child* within. Alternatively, our id can be understood in terms of the *devil* inside.

Our *super-ego* serves a role as our *conscience*. The super-ego aims for perfection and punishes misbehavior with guilt. Alternatively, the super-ego can be construed as the *angel* within us.

This framework of the psyche can be helpful in analyzing eating behaviors. Our eating can be *id-driven* in which we seek to achieve immediate pleasure and gratification with no thought of responsibility or of the long-term effects of that indulgence, a devil-may-care attitude. By the same token, *super-ego-driven* eating demands careful scrutiny and deliberation about any food item that is consumed, with great consideration given to mindful eating for the purpose of satisfying hunger and maintaining health. Any transgression from the super-ego's tight rein and control over eating behavior would result in guilt, the avoidance of which motivates angelic eating patterns. *Ego-driven* eating is the compromise between these two polar extremes. This is human eating behavior practiced by many of the one-third of the population that maintain a healthy weight—generally sensible, but with occasional excursions into id domain and super-ego domain that allow us to tip over into over-indulgent eating and then right ourselves.

Although some of us display primarily ego-driven eating with forays into id-driven eating that are checked by our super-ego drives, many of us are id-predominant and a few of us are super-ego-predominant. Those who do most of their eating based upon sheer instinct, with immediate-gratification-seeking consumption with no thought given to long-term consequences, are likely to be overweight or obese. Conversely, those whose eating style is tightly controlled and carefully measured, with the utmost of mindfulness applied to food choices and eating behavior, are unlikely to be overweight or obese. Super-ego-driven eating is not necessarily a healthy behavior—it can be extreme just as id-driven eating is—and its obsessive nature can lead to problems such as anorexia.

Another name for id-driven eating is promiscuous eating. This wanton, impulsive and reckless eating behavior can cause or contribute to obesity. A realistic goal to counteract id-driven promiscuous eating is to employ a mindful eating strategy in order to achieve balance and moderation—not obsessive mindfulness, simply a judicious amount of attention and awareness applied to our eating. We do not need to be angels at all moments! We simply need to be mindful of when and why the devil is influencing our behavior—be aware of it, think about it, understand it—and then either avoid the behavior, intervene by stopping before it gets out of hand or, if we must succumb, substituting a healthy alternative for an unhealthy indulgence. In other words, when our eating is id-driven, we should strive to recognize what is going on through mindfulness, and then turn on the super-ego to get us back on track to ego-driven eating.

Pavlov

Ivan Pavlov was a Russian physician, physiologist and psychologist who won the Nobel Prize in medicine. He is best known for describing *classical conditioning*, summarized as follows: meat causes dogs to salivate, an instinctual reaction called an *unconditioned response*. Pavlov used a metronome to call his dogs to their meaty meal and, after a few cycles of repetition, the dogs began to salivate on the basis of just the sound of the metronome. The reaction to the metronome is called a *conditioned response*, since it is a learned behavior.

Human beings are not all that different from Pavlov's dogs. Many foods literally elicit a "mouth watering" unconditioned response and certain specific contexts and environments can exact a conditioned response in the absence of the specific food item. This can certainly help explain the foraging for food that many of us pursue coincident with the television getting turned on. The same phenomenon happens in many movie theatres where accessory eating occurs as a result of the collusion of classical conditioning and opportunistic, temptation, and social forces. A similar situation happens to many of us as we enter our homes and head into the kitchen where all the food-associated context clues—the refrigerator, pantry, kitchen table, cookie jar, etc.—trigger our desire to eat via the classical conditioning pathway. The importance of classical conditioning vis-à-vis eating is that food-associated context cues can elicit a conditioned response that can trigger eating and drive overeating, weight gain and obesity.

A solution to eating driven by classical conditioning is to try to override it via mindfulness. When context is the initial drive to partake, the indulgence will not occur until the impulse becomes an action. When the television goes on and we get that strong urge to munch, in spite of not being hungry and perhaps just having finished a satisfying dinner, there are a number of solutions. We are intelligent and highly evolved cognitively, and we can and should be aware of the situation at hand. Before transforming the notion into an action, we can exercise a thought process to try to quell the conditioned response. That process might be musing about the folly of eating when not hungry, consideration of obesity, heart disease, clothes not fitting, flab around the waistline, etc. Our mindfulness and cognitive powers can override urges and reflexes—you might call this a mindful de-conditioning of a conditioned response.

Alternatively, we can succumb to the conditioned response, but eat only a small portion of the item we desire, or even better, swap our craving from its intended source to a healthy, colorful, crunchy, natural substitute such as fruit or veggies. Not only can we de-condition a conditioned response, but we also can actually re-condition ourselves to have a yearning for something healthy when we are exposed to context clues. Another possibility is to exchange the act of eating for an alternative activity such as exercising. An example of this is my post-work routine: after a day at the office, when I enter my house through the kitchen, I have conditioned myself to think of heading down to the basement to work out in lieu of staying in the kitchen and snacking.

Skinner

As a behavioral psychologist, B.F. Skinner believed that behavior could be explained on the basis of external and observable causes, and not by internal motivations. *Operant conditioning* is a means of learning governed by rewards and punishments meted out for the performance of certain behaviors. Behavioral change or learning occurs as associations are made between a given behavior and a consequence for that behavior. In operant conditioning, the promise or possibility of reward causes an increase in the behavior and the imposition of punishment causes a decrease of the behavior.

How does this relate to eating issues? For many of us, food functions to placate our state of emotional un-wellness. Comfort food consumption soothes our souls and drives continued comfort food consumption. *I'm really stressed and beaten up from a horrible day at work, so two large pieces of seven-layer chocolate cake are going to do the trick. I deserve it.* The problem is that this consumption is a behavior that begs repeating the next time the negative emotion surfaces. So, as the behavior gets reinforced again and again, a behavioral pattern gets established and over time, it gets more and more difficult to break. This is the very cycle of prompt-impulse-action-compensation-behavioral pattern discussed earlier. Additionally, food can serve as a reward for certain behaviors—*I did this, so I deserve that* kind of logic. *I passed the exam, so I deserve a hot fudge ice cream sundae.* So food serves a role in an entire range of emotional circumstances—to tranquilize and mollify a negative state, or, just as likely, to reward a positive state.

How do we combat the reward effect provided by the consumption of food to help calm our frazzled or heightened emotions? We must use Skinner's behavioral schema and *think* about the reward in *negative* terms—by mindful consideration of the long-term negative consequences of the continued behavioral pattern (being overweight, obese, diabetic, etc.) vs. the short-term reward/gain. Instead of a reward (*present*), we need to think *presence* of mind. The seeming reward is, in fact, a *punishment* to our long-term physical and emotional well being and serves only as a short term palliation that also functions to further perpetuate the cycle. Remember, in operant conditioning the promise or possibility of reward causes an increase in the behavior and punishment causes a decrease of the behavior. So, we are applying mindfulness to Skinnerian logic to think of emotional eating in terms of punishment to cause a decrease in the behavior. If mindfulness and intellectualization are insufficient to stem the emotional or reward eating, alternatively, consumption of just a taste (portion control) of the comfort food or reward is one possibility, and another is swapping out the reward for a healthier substitute, like exercising.

Csiksczentmihalyi

Mihaly Csiksczentmihalyi is a psychologist who has written about the concept of *flow*—a zen-like, heightened state of intention, concentration and complete mental engagement. This condition of full immersion in the activity at hand puts us *in the zone* where there are no distractions, time seemingly is arrested, our performance is optimal and a sense of fulfillment is derived. Achieving this state of *flow* requires focused attention and awareness, and pursuits including yoga, meditation and martial arts can help direct us into the flow groove.

To what extent flow can be cultivated is uncertain, although engaging in the aforementioned activities can definitely improve our abilities to become more mindful, which is a solid step towards achieving flow. It would seem that achieving the state of flow is equivalent to the ultimate state of mindfulness, *uber-mindfulness*, if you will. Mindfulness, awareness and attempts to achieve flow are powerful weapons when brought to the food and eating arena. With laser-focused mindfulness, dysfunctional eating patterns become more obvious and solutions more readily employed.

Proust

Marcel Proust was a French author who is known for his novel *Remembrance of Things Past*, in which it is revealed how the act of eating a madeleine pastry enables the narrator to evoke powerful memories with astonishing clarity and richness. Mere words cannot do justice to the remarkably vivid memories elicited and rekindled by the sight, smell and taste of this pastry, so the reader is referred to Proust's novel.

My personal "Proustian Madeleine" is a peach. When I grasp a fuzzy peach in my hand and draw it up to my face and breathe in deeply to take in the sweet aroma, I am immediately transported to the backyard of my grandparents' house. I am about ten years old and it is the peak of summer, the sun is high in the sky on an intensely blue-skied, cloudless day and verdant grass and shrubs surround my grandmother and me. Their neighbors have a grand old peach tree whose branches hang over into my grandparents' backyard. Many of the peaches are ripe and the air is redolent with the perfume of peaches ready to be eaten. I reach up and pick a big, perfectly round, pink and orange colored, downy, fragrant fruit. I bite into the succulent peach, close my eyes and the juice trickles down my face. When I open my eyes, my grandmother is smiling at my delight.

To this day, peaches evoke so many rich and vivid memories—times when there were no worries or responsibilities; my long since deceased, beloved grandmother; the warmth of summer; being outdoors on an idyllic day; nature; bliss. I am convinced that one of the reasons I love peaches, aside from the joy that they provide on face value, is their ability to allow me to revisit powerful memories and associations.

In essence, I have a deep-seated form of conditioned response to peaches—even sitting here at my computer engaged in writing on what happens to be a gray and sullen day, my thoughts are drawn to bright and vibrant summer memories, with greens and blues displacing the grays. My conditioned response of sorts is also an operant reward—a positive memory—from the thought process stirred up. This cheerful and upbeat conditioned response and operant reward will certainly drive me to continue to seek out peaches in particular, certainly a healthy indulgence. And I suppose that if it were a madeleine, a doughnut, or cheesecake that was the food item that evoked such happy memories, then I would be driven to eat them as opposed to my healthier indulgence.

Perhaps on a subconscious level, we are driven to eat food items that evoke in us a Proustian madeleine-type response and this may help explain in some way our propensity towards certain foods, whether they be healthy or not. Possibly, this may be a factor in the over-indulgence of certain food items that contribute to the American overweight and obesity epidemic. The Proustian response is such a formidable and compelling force that, if the food item that elicits the response is unhealthy, I am not sure that there is any simple solution. And if our positive Proustian moments are associated with healthy foods, we are most fortunate indeed.

CHAPTER 5

Solutions

Chew Over These Ideas

If I can claim it, it is mine. If I declare it, it has lost its power over me. Say your weak things in a strong voice.

Carrie Fisher, actress and author

Justin, age 35

I eat meal to meal—I do not think "big picture"—I try to make good choices versus poor choices without planning ahead.

The Battle of the Bulge

All right, enough psycho-chatter—let's get to business. Forget the theories, let us now be totally practical and get down to brass tacks and discuss solutions to the battle of the bulge. This will often require nothing short of donning our armor, planning offensive and defensive strategies, and getting battle-ready to combat the enemy. I will be borrowing a number of useful terms from military jargon that will be scattered throughout this chapter.

On the subject of the military, a panel of retired military leaders recently estimated that more than one quarter of potential 17- to 24-year-old recruits are too overweight to enlist in the armed forces. Because of their "too fat to fight" status, this panel appealed to Congress to eliminate junk foods and high-calorie beverages from schools, increase funding for healthy school lunches and endorse healthier lifestyles.

I use *tactic* to mean a plan for promoting a desired result; tactics are a *small picture* perspective focusing on the "trees" but not the "forest." I define *strategy* as a plan, method, or series of maneuvers and tactics for obtaining a specific goal or result; it is a *big picture* perspective that focuses upon the "forest" and not the "trees." Our ultimate goal is to improve our relationship with food and, in so doing, to achieve and maintain a healthy weight that will support our good health. By combining a number of different tactics that approach the battle from different angles and perspectives, we will be able to develop a strategy that can ultimately lead to life-long solutions.

It should be clear by now that emotional eating does not provide a long-term solution to our problems, but only a temporary, short-lived fix—if that—but it does indeed contribute to new stresses and a whole host of long-term health problems including obesity, hypertension, diabetes, cardiovascular diseases, cancer, etc. Unfortunately, the stress or other emotion that prompted the eating is still likely to be there the next day. To quote Roseanne Roseannadanna (the Saturday Night Live character played by Gilda Radner): *"It's always something—if it's not one thing, it's another"*! Ain't that the truth? Isn't there always some SNAFU (acronym for Situation Normal, All Fouled Up—or substitute an alternative "F" word!), getting in the way of the smooth sailing of our day-to-day existence? Life, for nearly all of us is often *complicated* and *difficult*, and overeating as a response is *easy*, but is neither an appropriate nor a healthy solution. In the battle against emotional eating or, for that matter, overeating for any reason, we need to understand *why* the behavior occurs and *address* the root cause appropriately. If there is no real solution to the underlying root cause, we at least need to be able to *manage* the problem with a coping mechanism that will not contribute negatively to our health. In other words, emotional eating often acts as a band-aid and not a long-term solution, and if there is no conceivable long-term solution, then a better band-aid—one that is not unhealthy—is in order.

At the vanguard of the conflict between basic eating drives and restraint is our highly evolved cerebral cortex that provides us with the capacity for mindfulness—knowledge of the salutary effects of maintaining a healthy weight and the unhealthy effects of excessive eating; understanding calories, energy expenditure, nutrition, which foods are healthy and which are not and how to read nutritional labels; comprehension and awareness of the emotions that drive our appetites; and the sensibility of when to stop eating by being in touch with our bodies. Mindfulness allows us to modulate our pleasure-pursuing and emotion-calming drives with restraint, overriding our potentially indulgent behaviors. When the eating-impelling forces predominate over the restraint forces, eating will inevitably occur and can help explain why intelligent people who know better cannot maintain a healthy weight.

We are privileged with the gift of brainpower—the ability to reason and to be creative, thoughtful, intelligent and emotive—and that is just *individual* intelligence. The *collective* intelligence of mankind has allowed us to achieve unimaginable feats and accomplishments. With respect to eating well and eating right, it would seem that many of us have the best of intentions, but in the course of our days, "obstacles" arise that interfere with the realization of our objectives. There is absolutely no reason that we cannot focus our minds and direct our cognitive capacities towards the goal of mindful eating, as mindful focus is the best means we have of combating and countering the numerous forces and pressures that constrain our good intentions.

Two general types of solutions can be helpful in the campaign against overeating issues—*behavioral* and *cognitive* techniques. Behavioral principles are mechanistic and are based on the concept that we can be educated about our eating condition and dysfunctional habits and develop simple tactics and strategies to minimize or eliminate the problem and re-establish control. Cognitive principles, on the other hand, involve mindfulness, introspection, thought and *intel* to provide solutions. Mindfulness serves as a form of internal *reconnaissance*—a heart-to-heart with ourselves and a careful observation and inventory of our own behavior. Knowledge of what we are doing and why—easier said than done and demanding some reflection and contemplation—is of fundamental importance. We want to be able to profit from the experience of our own past actions and this necessitates a complete absence of amnesia concerning our prior behaviors and feelings.

It begs answering the following questions: *Why are we eating? What are we eating? When are we eating? Where are we eating? How are we eating? How much are we eating?* It will demand applying our intelligence, knowledge, will and focus to the matter at hand. In the idealistic, utopian world of healthy eating, the correct answers to these questions are the following:

Why are we eating? Because we are genuinely hungry and need to fuel and nourish ourselves to maintain our health and provide the energy to live.

What are we eating? Real foods that are unprocessed, high quality, nutritious, natural, robust and wholesome and that will serve to promote our health and wellness and help us to avoid preventable diseases. Ideally, we will be aware of the origin of our foods and mindful of the caloric and nutritional content.

When are we eating? When we are genuinely hungry, preferably not late in the evening or in the middle of the night!

Where are we eating? In the perfect world, in the designated eating area, which is usually the kitchen, dining room, or restaurant; ideally, eating should be the total focus and mindless munching while lying in bed reading, sitting in the chaise lounge watching television or while driving should be minimized. This is not to say that an occasional meal or snack should not be enjoyed while being entertained by the television or watching a movie.

How are we eating? In a slow and deliberate manner, taking the time to appreciate and savor the food and enjoy the moment.

How much are we eating? A reasonable and moderate serving that will satiate us without leaving us feeling full and bloated.

Tactics, Strategies and Solutions

The following pages will enumerate and explain a number of different approaches to winning the battle of the bulge, and in broader terms, winning the war on overeating, weight gain and obesity.

Be mindful of why we are hungry. It is of fundamental importance to learn the difference between when our hunger is on an emotional basis and when it is on a physical basis. Our goal should be to eat only when physically hungry, not when emotionally hungry. We must clearly understand that emotional factors—such as stress, fatigue, depression, mood swings, loneliness, boredom, feelings of deprivation, the need for immediate gratification, etc.—beg for a convenient and immediate source of relief and interfere with our mindfulness, which is our key asset in the fight against overeating.

It is important to pay attention to the specific emotional triggers that promote our self-destructive eating behaviors and to understand that when life leaves us feeling a sense of deprivation, that void cannot be effectively filled with food. We cannot eat food to gain self esteem—we will just end up gaining weight!

Mindfulness enables us to know what we are doing and why we are doing it to help determine the root cause of our behavior. Carefully keeping a food journal makes it easy to figure out the relationship between emotional triggers and the consumption of specific foods. Thereafter, we need to deal with the underlying cause in as productive a means as possible. If the root cause cannot be conquered—which is often the case as there is no end to the degree, range and variety of emotional reactions to what life brings us— then we need to learn a more appropriate means of handling our response to the emotion via techniques such as food swapping and activity swapping.

Use the buddy system. When we were children, we used this system to ensure our safety when swimming. Our "buddy" was on the lookout for us. In similar fashion, the *buddy system*, an extension of "it takes a village," can be of great help to us in the eating domain. Essentially, this involves a family member or friend being on our team to help us out at times of weakness. When they observe us eating "inappropriately," they can offer constructive criticism to set us back on the right track.

One evening I was watching television with my family and found myself exhausted and dozing off. After the movie ended around 11PM, I headed to the kitchen to toast whole wheat bread and melt some cheese on top. My wife saw me about to succumb to "fatigue eating" and stopped me, suggesting that I head up to bed and that I would be unhappy with myself in the morning for indulging in unnecessary late night eating not driven by hunger. She was absolutely right and I woke up in the morning with no regrets.

Keep a food journal. This is a simple way of documenting what we eat on any given day and sometimes the results are astonishing, demonstrating a great discrepancy between our perception of what we eat and what we actually do eat. Additionally, it is a nice means of ascertaining the relationship between our emotions and what we eat, delineating when or what situations drive the eating behavior and which foods cause mood swings, improve our emotional state, etc. A food journal is a valuable tool that costs nothing and certainly will help hone our mindfulness and self-awareness, and ultimately will aid in improving our eating habits. *Personal-nutrition-guide.com* offers a fabulous, free, downloadable "Food'n'Mood Journal." It is best to keep a record for one week, one day at a time. The following parameters are recorded: time, place, food/beverage consumed, quantity, mood before eating, mood after eating.

Food swapping is a very utilitarian means of substituting a healthy, low-calorie food for an indulgence that is likely laden in calories, fat, sugar and salt. So, instead of us eating a plate of nachos while watching a rental movie, we can substitute a nice fruit plate. This exchange can result in satisfaction without the calories, guilt and remorse that can ensue from many indulgences. If it is alcohol that prompts the excessive eating, then a non-alcoholic beverage that still retains the taste, such as non-alcoholic beer or wine, is a consideration.

Activity swapping is a constructive maneuver in which eating behavior that is driven by emotional impulses is exchanged for an alternative behavior that has an equivalent soothing effect. This substitute activity for eating might be sleep, exercise, reading, phoning a friend, getting out of our home, taking a walk, taking a bath or shower, doing household work or errands—anything to get our minds off the craving. When fatigue drives eating, obviously taking a nap or getting some sleep is of utility and addresses the matter at hand. When it is stress or anxiety that precipitates the eating, exercise, yoga, meditation or other relaxation techniques can be particularly productive alternative activities that work. Healthy means of stress management also include massages, getting into a jacuzzi, aromatherapy, chamomile or other herbal teas, etc. Let us not forget about sex as a wonderful means of stress relief! When it is boredom or the need for immediate gratification that prompts the eating, it is simply a question of finding a suitable substitute endeavor, hobby, or interest that will be a less caloric activity than eating—gardening, woodworking, painting, knitting, whatever. The swapped activity must be reasonable and not one that ultimately engenders stress—for example, someone I know shops as an alternative to eating, but when the large credit card bills arrive, she has even more "new" stress than the "original" stress.

Alicia, age 54

I conquer boredom grazing with a substitute activity such as crocheting.

Diana, age 26

When angry or stressed, I deal with it by cleaning or folding up the laundry. When my job was on the line, I purposely stockpiled the laundry, knowing that it would come in handy.

Paulina, age 49

I used to eat because of boredom. I would get home from work at 3PM, but my husband would not come home until 6PM, so I would have a cocktail with chips, nachos, cheese, and some cookies. I joined a gym, so now I exercise instead of drinking cocktails and eating food. Now that I am working out, I find that I am consuming fewer carbohydrates and am better at portion control.

Mind portions. Portion control is of fundamental importance for anyone and everyone who wants to achieve a desirable weight. This is, perhaps, the greatest asset that we can "bring to the table" no matter what the cause of the overeating. More calories in than out equals weight gain—fewer calories in than out equals weight loss. Whether we have satiety issues and do not feel as full as we think we should, or whether we are eating for emotional reasons, or if we desire to lose weight for any reason, one of the key elements is mindful apportioning of foods and stopping after appropriate caloric consumption. It is a smart tactic for us to decide at the beginning of any meal precisely how much we are going to consume and, if possible, place everything we plan on eating on our plate and eat that and only that. As an alternative to the one-plate idea, another tactic is to serve high-calorie foods directly on our plates and low-calorie items like vegetables on the table, family-style.

So, whether we are impelled to eat for hunger or for emotional reasons, we need to be attentive to the situation at hand and eat reasonably and, if possible, to make an effort to consume healthy foods. If we do fall prey to mindless eating, we should be *mindfully* mindless enough to be moderate in our consumption. One of the people I interviewed referred to this as "portion-controlled emotional eating."

Another advantage of portion control is that the decreased food consumption results in more resources that can go towards purchasing higher quality, healthier, locally grown foods.

Portions are very much influenced by the *size* of snack packages, plates, bowls, utensils, etc., with the larger the plate, the deeper the bowl, the bigger the bag, the more we tend to eat. The small plate trick is really a very good one—psychology playing a profound effect on our eating behaviors—a very full but small plate that contains less food than a partially full but larger plate will often seem to have more food and be equally, if not more, filling. It is a prudent idea to try and not eat directly from a package, but to apportion out a serving, simply because the bag is a "black hole" and most of us have no idea of the portion that we ultimately consume as our hands go from bag to mouth, again and again (unless of course, the entire bag is consumed, a very real possibility!). Using small utensils—particularly forks and spoons—will not only slow us down, but will also create the illusion that we are eating more. Another effective tactic to slow down our eating is to use chopsticks as utensils!

When dining out, it is a sensible idea to share entrees or order an appetizer for an entree. When it comes time for dessert, certainly a taste will do, won't it? We have already probably consumed an oversized meal, likely of greater volume and higher in calories than we would have at home, and we are simply in search of a novel taste to serve as the grand finale for the meal. We should not eat dessert to be filled up, but simply for a concluding piquing and titillation of our taste buds.

Kyle, age 44

On Thursday evenings I play soccer, then go out drinking with the boys. I have a few vodkas, which tends to make me want to eat even though I am not hungry. I will order wings or a sample platter. Sometimes I just eat the celery or maybe dip it in hot sauce with a little blue cheese. I try not to eat fast foods or junk—if I want chips, I will eat three.

Alicia, age 54

After overindulging, I feel guilty, bad, horrible, but I accept my emotional eating as long as I exercise portion control.

Mind the calories. I do not espouse weighing our food on a scale, nor counting every calorie with the demeanor of an accountant; however, it is important to have a general sense of how many calories a particular food item has. This is becoming much easier because of improved nutritional labels and more nutritional "transparency"; as part of the health care legislation that was signed into law in 2010, every big restaurant chain in the nation is now required to post calorie information on their menus and drive-through signs.

It is important to understand the discrepancy between the caloric content of a "serving" as defined on the nutritional label of a packaged food item and the actual calories of the "serving" that we dole out for ourselves. In many instances, our concept of a serving is at great odds with the actual serving size recommended on the box, and we end up consuming many more calories than we think we are. This is especially true of cereals and pastas.

It is also rather beneficial to have a general sense of caloric expenditure with exercise, so we can get a concept of how much exercise it takes to burn off a caloric load. This information can be invaluable in terms of its ability to influence our food choices.

Last evening I was in Starbucks with my wife and we ordered coffees and shared a piece of "reduced fat very berry cake." This relatively thin slice had 350 calories, knowledge gleaned from the mandate that chain restaurants with more than 15 locations nationwide must list calorie counts on their menu boards. Knowing the precise calorie count was very sobering information and having access to this certainly influenced me to carefully consider what I chose to eat and how much I decided to eat. Realizing that 350 calories is about the equivalent of running 3.5 miles put a damper on my consumption!

Kyle, age 44

I find the Live Strong calorie tracker that I use on my iPod Touch phone to be very useful.

Mind how we eat. It is important to eat slowly and deliberately with the endpoint of achieving satiety and not fullness. Mindlessly munching away at our meals or eating like a starved hyena is clearly not our goal. Eating at a leisurely pace, mindfully and attentively, and taking the time to see, smell, hear, touch, and taste food, enjoying the experience and appreciating the moment is our goal.

If we have become habituated to eating to the point of feeling stuffed and even physically uncomfortable, our stomachs will gradually stretch out over time to accommodate this, creating a vicious cycle in which more volume is needed to achieve that feeling of fullness that we have come to desire. More volume equals more calories equals more weight gain. So the goal is not to devour, gorge and overindulge, but to enjoy the process and stop when satiety and satisfaction are achieved. There is a delay period between food intake and the feeling of satiety, so slow and measured eating will get us to that point with less volume of food consumed and thus less of a caloric load.

Ideally, we should avoid family style dining and apportion *one* nice plate of food—certainly sufficient and reasonable in terms of nourishment and ability to quell hunger—and understand at the outset that that is the meal, the whole meal, the entire meal, so it needs to be eaten slowly and savored to make it last. We should remember to load the plate up with healthy, high-fiber, low-calorie veggies. We need to take reasonable bites, not shovelfuls, chew slowly, take some "time-outs" and sit back and enjoy. It is always a good idea to put down our utensils between bites and engage in a good conversation if possible, since eating is a wonderful social activity. It is reasonable after putting down our forks to not pick them up until the bite is swallowed.

Foods that are very hot (tea and soup for example), or very cold (deeply frozen ice cream), can only be consumed at a very slow pace to avoid getting burned and to avoid "brain freeze," respectively. Just as we can only *sip* hot liquids and only eat something rock-frozen very slowly, so should this eating style be applied to eating *anything*. If we suffer from turbo-guzzling, it behooves us to opt for the types of foods that just cannot be eaten in this manner—foods that are naturally more difficult to eat rapidly because they require work.

Eat as our cells eat. Our body consists of *organs*, the organs are made of *tissues* and the tissues consist of *cells*. Our cells are in need of energy to run, but energy in very controlled and small amounts. The energy currency of our cells is ATP, a molecule of adenosine bound to three phosphates. It takes extra energy to bind the second to the third phosphate and this provides the source of power for our cells. When our cells need energy, the ATP is broken down into ADP, releasing the third phosphate and a burst of energy. So ATP can be thought of as a fully charged battery and ADP as the spent battery.

The energy derived from our diet is in the form of calories from carbohydrates, fats, and proteins. These macronutrients are the fodder for replenishing our ATP batteries. A large meal cannot be burned all at once like kindling on a fire, since this would not be useful in terms of our cells, which are in constant need of energy in controlled, constant and minute amounts. In terms of providing the energy necessary for our metabolism, *eating as our cells eat* means the consumption of frequent, small meals. This is a very physiological and healthy manner of eating, although there is certainly nothing wrong with the traditional three meals per day eating style. "Grazing" does not allow our stomachs to get so over-stuffed and stretched that satiety issues can occur over the long-term.

This grazing style of eating is not unlike how we take frequent sips of water when we are exercising to satisfy our thirst and prevent dehydration. Many weight loss experts often promote grazing insofar as people who eat in this way find themselves generally less hungry and more energized since their metabolisms are receiving continual small "boosts." Remember that the potential exists to abuse grazing—if we over-graze, we can wind up eating more food than we would have if we ate the standard three meals with some snacking!

Kirsten, age 31

I am a grazer who wants a small taste of everything. I eat half entrees; I always try to cut meals in half or have an appetizer instead of an entree. I rarely overeat, but if I do so, I don't feel well at all.

It is not a good idea to skip meals. It is unhealthy, it is not eating as our cells eat, and it can promote over-compensation from the rebound hunger and desire to make up for the caloric deprivation. Granted, some of us are not very hungry at certain times of the day.

I, for one, do not have much of an appetite for breakfast and often find myself eating not to satisfy hunger but to provide myself with the proper nutrition and calories (plus caffeine I must add), to start my day with a bang after what effectively amounts to a twelve or more hour fast.

John, age 26

I skip a lot of meals and often don't eat until later afternoon—then I eat way too much and way too fast—if I pace myself, it helps a lot. When I haven't eaten until 4 or 5PM I get excited thinking that I am owed something indulgent—that I have "saved up my money in the bank" and that I am owed something really good.

Avoid late night eating. Eating near sleep time is an extremely bad habit that contributes to weight gain, insomnia and guilt. Sleep is the most metabolically dormant time of the day for us, so the consumption of large amounts of food late at night, particularly right before going to sleep, will provide us with a large caloric load at a time when we burn the least amount of calories. It is the equivalent of pumping our cars full of fuel only to store them in the garage. Additionally, the bloating and intestinal stimulation can interfere with our achieving a good night's sleep, and we know how fatigue can further exacerbate our eating tendencies. It is an abysmal feeling to awaken in the morning feeling bloated, flabby and guilty as a result of the unnecessary and promiscuous consumption of food. Starting a new day feeling emotionally, mentally, and physically compromised because of late night bingeing is a situation that might be referred to in military jargon as FUBAR—Fouled Up Beyond All Recognition (or substitute an alternative F word!).

I make an effort to let the last thing I eat before heading off to bed be natural and healthy—such as a piece of fruit; by finishing off the day on a nutritious note, it allows one to start the next day feeling physically and emotionally spirited.

John, age 26

If I eat a big meal really late, I feel awful, bloated and disgusted when I wake up in the morning; however, if I eat something like oatmeal with a banana, I feel great.

Sleep the calories away. Adequate quantity and quality of sleep is of obvious importance to our general well being and optimal functioning. We have all enjoyed the blissful experience of a great night's sleep, in which we awaken feeling rested, energetic, optimistic and ready to tackle the new day with vigor. Conversely, we have all experienced a very poor night's sleep, in which we awaken feeling physically exhausted, mentally spent, lids heavy, dark circles under our eyes and in a disassociated "zombie" state, totally unprepared and unenthusiastic about facing the new day. Sleeping has a vitally important restorative function—our batteries need to be recharged—our brains and bodies require this important down time. Insufficient sleep results in decreased levels of *leptin* (our chemical appetite suppressant), increased *ghrelin* levels (our chemical appetite stimulant), increased *corticosteroids* (stress hormones), and increased *glucose* levels (higher amounts of sugar in the bloodstream). Acute sleep disruption is associated with increased appetite and caloric intake and chronic sleep deficits result in an inability to be attentive and focused, interfering with our mindfulness, which can further wreak havoc with our eating. The disassociated "zombie" state lends itself to dysfunctional eating patterns and, as such, weight gain is a predictable consequence. A chronically fatigued state also will affect our ability to exercise properly, if at all.

Designate an eating area. We exercise in the basement, we shower in the bathroom, we sleep in the bedroom, and ideally we should eat in the designated eating area of our homes, which is usually the kitchen or dining room. We tend to get into trouble when we eat in our bedrooms, living rooms, cars, desks at work, and so forth. When we eat, we should really make every effort to give it our undivided attention—when eating is one of our activities when multi-tasking, mindless and excessive consumption is the usual outcome. This is why eating while reading, watching television, talking on the telephone, checking our e-mail, etc., is so dangerous.

Katherine, age 56

Because of my OCD, I never eat anywhere but the kitchen, because I don't want to get crumbs in the living room. So, to this day, neither my children nor I eat while watching television.

Jacqueline, age 19
I eat when I am distracted, for example, when I watch television.

Amy, age 62
I don't eat while watching television since I am so focused on what I am watching.

Mind the trigger foods that drive overeating. For many of us, it is the refined "white" carbohydrates with their addictive properties that can precipitate and engender a vicious cycle of overeating. Worth reiterating is the fact that processed wheat is so addictive because the grain is hulled and stripped of the bran and germ, resulting in a pulverized, super-fine, silky white powder. This highly refined substance is very similar in appearance to cocaine or heroin and this pre-chewed-pre-digested-melts-in-your-mouth-adult-baby-food equivalent is so rapidly transformed into glucose and absorbed that it is similar to getting an injection of glucose intravenously. This *quick fix* is not filling because of the absence of fiber—it is a short-lived satisfaction that begs for more consumption, establishing a vicious cycle. Once we recognize what foods spark the behavior we wish to avoid, it then becomes a matter of minimizing our exposure to them. This is more easily said than done, but is an important first step on the pathway that we seek to travel on.

Many of those who are addicted to trigger foods literally cannot have *any* exposure to these foods, lest they sabotage themselves and fall into a downward spiral of overeating and weight gain. Conceptually similar to an alcoholic or drug addict, the food addict must simply practice abstinence. If a "white carb" addict has a "taste" of their trigger food, what they are really doing to themselves is what in military jargon is BOHICA, an acronym for Bend Over, Here It Comes Again!

It is very interesting that many of those I interviewed clearly stated that when liberated from their addictive trigger foods, they not only lose their urges and desires for them, but the very thought of the foods in question can actually be repugnant.

Vanessa, age 47

My downfall is white carbs, to which I am addicted. Once I get started, I literally cannot stop. If I have a bagel, I will need to continue eating bagels. I have come to the realization that white carbs physically and mentally make me feel like crap—tired, fatigued, and lacking energy. Proteins and fats satisfy my appetite and don't leave me feeling like white carbs do. I have had yo-yo weight issues for years and have been on Weight Watchers four or five times, Nutrasystem, and the South Beach diet. For me, the South Beach diet works best, because of the limitation on carbohydrates, which are my trigger foods, and the fact that I don't have to measure portions, which I loathe.

Talia, age 56

I am addicted to sweets. When I lost 20 lbs for my son's wedding, my sugar craving largely disappeared.

Break our ingrained dysfunctional eating habits. We are humans and have developed many habitual behaviors, some of which are good, some of which are bad. Many of us have deeply ingrained, highly reinforced, dysfunctional eating habits that contribute to our weight issues. Pretty much anytime we eat while participating in other activities is indicative of a bad eating habit—for example, eating while driving, cooking, reading, watching television, talking on the telephone, etc.

We must first identify the habit, recognize why it is dysfunctional and instrumental to our weight problem, and then make an effort to break the habit. Breaking entrenched and deep-rooted habits does not come easily or readily. Resisting temptation is very difficult, but if triumphant the first time, each successive effort at resistance becomes that much easier. Sometimes, developing *new habits* via repetition can be helpful—for example, instead of entering our homes through the kitchen, we can come in through another door and simply avoid the room where the contextual cues trigger our eating. Alternatively, we can cultivate the habit of exercising when we get home from work. When all else fails, we can food swap for a healthy substitute when we cannot avoid the temptation to eat when participating in other activities—carrot sticks instead of chips will incur a lot less harm to us when we are compelled to "multi-task" consume.

Jonathon, age 52

I am accustomed to being a "night nosher," although my eating during the day is very controlled. As soon as I get home, I have to have a snack. Then I eat a good dinner, which satisfies my appetite. Right after dinner, I start grazing. Even though I am in another room and not hungry, I will head into the kitchen and grab some peanuts, raisins, and maybe a slice or two of turkey. Once I start with one thing, it leads to another.

Drink plenty of fluids, but don't drink too many of our calories. At times, our bodies confuse thirst with hunger. I know for a fact that this happens to me and I have found that I have attempted to quell my thirst with eating—a behavior that is not a particularly efficient means of hydration, nor healthy in terms of the potential for gaining unnecessary pounds. Drinking good old water will do the trick in terms of maintaining our hydration, at a cost of zero calories. This is in comparison to sodas—carbohydrate-laden empty calories typically sweetened with high fructose corn syrup—essentially liquid candy.

After an exercise session, even though I have tried to maintain my hydration with water consumption during the workout, I find that I have a profound "appetite." Often, by drinking something more substantive than water, but healthy—for example, carrot juice, kefir (a rich, yogurt-like drink) or a fruit shake—I find that my "appetite" is truly slaked.

I enjoy fruit smoothies made with fat-free milk or soy milk, fat-free yogurt and fruit, particularly after exercising. I keep a bag of mixed frozen fruit in the freezer just for this purpose, which is especially useful during the winter months when fresh fruit is less available in the northeastern United States. It is extremely filling and refreshing, quenches my thirst and cools me down after a long bike ride or good workout. It is low in calories, has no fat, contains plenty of protein and carbohydrates, is chock full of antioxidants, and is very filling. I use a variety of different fruits to shake it up. I try all sorts of

combinations, most recently fresh blackberries, strawberries, blueber-
ries, raspberries and bananas, which turned out to be a particularly
delicious combination. Even my kids enjoy these, and they are a whole
lot healthier than the mixed concoctions you buy at the mall.

Jonathon, age 52
I find that if I drink a few glasses of water before a meal, I will end up eating less.

Access control is a helpful tactic because of the simple reason that
whatever is handy is readily eaten and whatever is not handy is not
readily eaten. In other words, *in sight* leads to a greater chance of
consumption, hungry or not! Out of sight, out of mind, so we ought
to try to keep junk or trigger foods stashed away or unavailable. This
is the equivalent of a *preemptive strike,* which I define as an attack
made upon the enemy—addictive trigger foods—as a precautionary
response to an anticipated or impending battle.

By keeping fruits and vegetables easily accessible—such as a
bowl of fresh fruit left on the counter in the kitchen and cut up fresh
vegetables ready for consumption in the refrigerator—we are making
them available, which will likely lead to their consumption instead
of unhealthier foods that are made less accessible. As humans, we
are *very* susceptible to advertising, and just the act of looking at a
food item draws our attention to it and often entices us. Out of sight
also means storing less desirable food items in opaque as opposed
to transparent containers or on higher shelves that are difficult to
reach. Ideally, unhealthy foods should not be available in the house
at all.

Controlling access is a behavioral technique that can help the
process of weight management, but is not the absolute solution since
the ultimate means of controlling access is our *mindfulness*, which
if cultivated sufficiently, should allow us control even in the face of
ample opportunity for over-indulgence—and this is the ultimate goal
since we cannot always control our environment. So, the quintessential safe haven from opportunistic eating lies within us—couched
inside our cranial bones—wherever we go, we bring with us our pre-
cious mind, that when turned on full-throttle should allow us to control ourselves in the midst of opportunity and temptation. We need

to be able to trust ourselves around food and in order to avoid a sense of self-deprivation, we need to be able to exist among the presence of all foods.

If we find that controlling access to food is of paramount help in terms of watching our caloric intake, then certain venues should probably be actively avoided. One of these is cruise vacations, where five huge meals are served daily, food is available 24/7, and where a major focus of the entertainment is actually dining. Another is all-you-can-eat venues, such as Chinese buffets, Brazilian barbecues, and other restaurants that offer this eating *bonanza* that really represents a *burden*. For many of us, *any* restaurant can represent a challenge to our weight management, since there are so many unknowns in terms of caloric and nutritional content, as well as open-ended opportunity, the social environment and alcohol, all factors that can spur overeating.

Jackie, age 50
We order out a lot, which is a killer.

The following is one of the stories I found most entertaining . . . and most amazing, but true!

Gwen, age 63
When stressed or bored, I eat ice cream. I chip away at it in grazing-like fashion, but can polish off half a gallon. I do not get relief, only feel more stress and I vow I will be better tomorrow. I will then gather up all the junk foods in my house and toss them in the garbage. However, I have been known to take them right back out of the garbage. So I spray wasp repellant on the food in the trash, so that I will not take it out and eat it. I am usually good for a few weeks after this.

Wow . . . controlling access by plying unhealthy food with poison—if this is what it takes, go for it (just watch your children and pets)!

Accept and compensate is a pragmatic strategy when eating is inevitable for a variety of circumstances. Overeating may occur because of hormonal factors in a female prior to menstruation; because of seasonal factors such as the short, cold days of winter; when mindfulness cannot override the drive to eat on an emotional basis; or under circumstances of socialized, conditioned, opportunistic eating such as in movie theatres, while watching television or sporting events or attending celebrations or holiday meals. Accept and compensate means that we willingly acquiesce to our eating desires but do so with the mindfulness to indulge in moderation, swap for a healthy alternative, or to make an effort to burn more calories with exercise or any kind of augmented physical activity. So, if push comes to shove and we must succumb to our compulsion to eat, under these circumstances, portion control rules. Ideally, this means *one* small plate filled with our craving.

Jacqueline, age 19

If I'm going to binge, I do healthy binge eating—strawberries and raw vegetables.

Nicole, age 33

I was supposed to get a promotion and raise but didn't, so I ate 3 chocolate chip cookies, which is a lot for me. I felt bad and compensated by being more aware the next day and upping my exercise, even if it was just moving about the house doing things.

When we overdo it with eating, break our diets, or succumb to emotional prompts, there are a number of ways to compensate for our behavior. We can exercise to burn off the excessive calories consumed. Alternatively, we can balance it out by eating less the following day. It is important to maintain a long-term perspective and simply accept the deviation for what it is—none of us being perfect—and resume a disciplined and mindful eating style, recognizing that a short-term over-indulgence is meaningless over the long-term. Going off the wagon via a temporary lapse of mindfulness does not mean that we need to resume a reckless pattern of mindless eating and self-destructive, self-loathing behavior. We can fall off for a moment, but climb right back on!

I had a ventral hernia repair that required me not to exercise for at least several weeks, a very troublesome and disturbing concept for a daily exerciser. My compensation was to further hone my already respectable eating habits. I decided that as long as I could not exercise,

I would make an effort to make every snack a healthy one. So, for example, one evening while watching some movies with my family (yes, I am guilty of media munching), I had a grapefruit, an apple and a bunch of baby carrots. No way was I letting my forced sabbatical from the exercise that I love to participate in ruin my overall fitness and wellness lifestyle!

Vaccinate and inoculate. We are accustomed to getting vaccinated and inoculated with a small dose of virus or bacteria to prevent an infection at a later date. The same concept can apply to eating. During the course of our days, many of us have numerous opportunities for food consumption, particularly at work, where there may be plenty of available and tempting food for the taking. It may be a colleague's birthday and a great big piece of birthday cake with gooey icing is sitting there, just begging to be consumed. What to do?

> Option #1: Enjoy the piece of cake, delight in the camaraderie and help your colleague celebrate. *The problem is that the cake is unhealthy and if we are concerned about our weight, it is definitely a poor choice.*

> Option #2: Decline the cake, demonstrating ferocious willpower and observe your colleagues joyfully devouring their pieces. *The problem with this approach is that it will likely make us feel a sense of deprivation and unfairness that just might backfire, resulting in us over-compensating later with an even higher caloric indulgence; plus, it tends to make us look like anti-social ascetics!*

> Option # 3: Vaccinate and inoculate—take a small piece, a teeny but satisfying taste, a vaccination if you will—a small dose that will preclude us from coming down with the disease— the obesity disease. *The benefit of this compromising approach is enjoying the moment and the camaraderie without deprivation, yet maintaining an overall healthy eating style by this very moderate indulgence.*

I found myself sitting in the lounge of the surgical center where I do most of my ambulatory surgery cases, having some free time between procedures. On the table were a couple of packages of chocolate rugelach that one of the anesthesiologists generously brought in. The pastries not only looked great, but also smelled delicious. I picked up the package and read the contents: bad-bad-bad in every respect. But opportunity and temptation knocked loudly, so even though I was not hungry, this most appealing sweet was sitting at arm's length away, begging me to indulge. So I caved in, brewed myself a cup of coffee and cut a very small piece of rugelach, perhaps a quarter of the pastry, and savored it with the coffee. Even though it was full of unhealthy processed junk, it was certainly not an over-indulgence by any measure and served to provide a nice, satisfying and delicious tasting snack, a fine complement to the coffee.

The moral of the story is that if we are going to engage in op-portunistic/temptation eating, by exercising some portion control, we are not going to do ourselves too much harm—and by having just a taste, we will prevent rebound over-indulgence. Everything in moderation, including moderation!

Justin, age 35

I believe in the occasional purposeful indulgence to prevent a major indulgence later—for me, a piece of dark chocolate or one scoop of ice cream, etc., does the trick.

Vaccinate and inoculate is a successful tactic for me, a real *coup*, if you will, but it will not be successful for everyone. There are some who have such a profound addiction to certain trigger foods that even a small exposure to that food can set off a cascading cycle that demands more and more of that particular food. For this subset of the population, total avoidance is the key, being similar to an alco-holic not being able to have even one drink.

Enjoy the olfactory experience. The pleasure of eating involves the stimulation of many senses simultaneously. Our sense of smell is a very important component of the pleasure derived from eating. Re-member how tasteless food becomes when we have a cold and nasal congestion. If we take a small taste of chocolate and then bring the empty wrapper to our noses and inhale deeply, we receive a blast of calorie-free chocolate aroma stimulation that is *almost* as good as eating the chocolate. For some, this might prove to be too much of a tease, but for many, a small taste supplemented with a brisk inhalation of the rich and intense scent can be very satisfying.

Bank and burn calories can be a very useful tactic when we anticipate being in a situation that will expose us to opportunistic eating or the potential for over-indulgence. Say, for example, that we plan on going to a celebration, a holiday dinner or on a vacation. Very simply, prior to our "event," we show caloric restraint (bank reduced caloric intake) and ramp up the exercise (burn) so that we can have a moderate over-indulgence and feel no remorse about it.

Carmen, age 18

I adore homemade chocolate ice cream with hot fudge, whipped cream, and chocolate shavings. When I know I will be splurging later, I will "pre-compensate" for the many calories I will be having by eating a few healthy meals before—for example, having fruit for lunch.

Kyle, age 44

I will be hosting a super bowl party so I will run in the morning to counterbalance my eating. This will make me feel less guilty. And if I do overeat, the next day I will eat less and make sure I get to the gym.

Stay busy and productive. So many of us, when engaged and occupied, do not even think about eating; in fact, when we are truly absorbed and immersed in the matter at hand, may forget to eat completely! Many of those I interviewed reported that their situation was well controlled during the day when busy and occupied at work, despite ample opportunity for temptation, but bad in the evening when home. Boredom is the devil when it comes to eating. So, a simple and effective means of weight management is to live a rich and full life with lots of activities to occupy ourselves with, such that eating becomes much less of a focus.

Writing this book was an extremely exciting and engaging process. It was so absorbing and captivating that I often found that time raced by and as mealtimes approached, I had a rather minimal appetite, a very strange phenomenon for me.

Amy, age 62

I have ample opportunity to eat while at work as we have a well-stocked coffee room with doughnuts, cakes, and bagels available. When tempted, I keep myself busy, and I forget all about eating.

Oral alternatives. Eating is all about oral stimulation. Chewing gum, sucking candy or breath mints can provide low-calorie oral stimulation that is an alternative to eating. If you keep your mouth occupied, then eating is precluded, so some other oral alternatives are engaging in a good conversation or singing.

Mindful snacking. Snacking is absolutely fine as long as we make every effort to eat nutritious snacks. Natural and unprocessed is best. Fresh fruit, fresh vegetables, nuts and dried fruit make great snacks that are satisfying, can quell our appetites, and the fiber content serves to fill us up and slow down the carbohydrate absorption. We must keep in mind the caloric density of dried fruits and nuts, so moderation needs to be exercised. A *few* pieces of dried fruit—including raisins, apricots, cranberries, figs, dates, prunes—or even fresh baby carrots are a nice alternative to non-nutritious, sugary snacks when we get a craving for something sweet.

Stephanie, age 52

I lost 100 lbs with the help of a diet doctor, medications and avoidance of carbohydrates. I used to eat when upset, stressed, or sad and would go for bagels, bread, cookies, and cake. I gave up emotional eating and pasta, potatoes, bread and other carbs. Now I snack on celery, carrots, and water.

Isabelle, age 10

I try to steer away from the food cabinet, but if I find myself there, I try to pick things that are not bad, but are not as good as fresh vegetables, an apple or organic food. So I will pick something like Goldfish baked snack crackers.

Exercise restraint. Yes, it is noble not to waste anything, particularly foods. At the same time, being the designated "clean up" person in your family—eating the kids' leftovers until their plates are squeegee clean, polishing off every last pizza crust or getting every morsel of flesh off the chicken bones and ribs in piranha-like fashion—is undesirable behavior and contributes to "the problem." We need to keep to our own plates and leave the leftovers for that friendly canine with his head on our laps.

As an exercise to our wills, we can make an effort to leave a bite or so of food left on our plates. Easier said than done, this exercise will help us eat to satiety and not to fullness and help many of us break the goal-oriented, finish-the-job style of eating that we are habituated to.

I am very much a goal-oriented individual who is in the habit of completing the task at hand, and I find that I bring this to the table in that I rarely leave any food on my plate, which is really not very wise! My wife knows that if there are any remains on my plate then I am either unwell or have been served a really super-sized portion.

Vittoria, age 50

I feel obligated to finish a sandwich even though I am full. My stomach ends up in my chest, I feel guilty, bloated and can't breathe.

Jonathon, age 52

My biggest issue is that I eat what is put in front of me. So I always try to take a little something away from what I'm eating. For example, at a restaurant I will remove one piece of bread from a sandwich, or if I'm making a sandwich, I will use two slices of turkey instead of three. At dinner, where I might eat two pieces of chicken, I will take one piece, cut it in half, and now have "two pieces."

Exercise to exorcise. Exercise is great in a multitude of ways and we do not need an expensive gym membership to participate. The real key is staying active, kinetic and moving. Exercise can be integrated into our daily activities—for example, gardening, snow shoveling, mowing the lawn, sawing tree branches, walking the dog, carrying a heavy laundry basket, vacuuming, taking out the recycling, carrying our child on our backs, dancing, etc. If possible, we can walk or bike to work instead of driving. We can also use the stairs instead of the elevator or the escalator. We can park far away from our intended destination at the mall, and burn calories and be good to our environment at the same time. We can play Wii-Fit with our children—it's really a great deal of fun!

Exercise burns calories, improves our strength and fitness and makes us feel energized. When our physical fitness improves, it seems to help inspire good eating habits. Equally so, good eating habits seem to inspire many of us to exercise. So, there seems to be some sort of synergism between exercise and healthy eating—healthy habits engender more healthy habits and unhealthy habits promote unhealthy habits. Many of those I interviewed reported that if they were actively engaged in some sort of exercise regimen on a regular basis, they were less likely to fall prey to bingeing provoked by emotional reasons, and that if they were not exercising, they were more likely to succumb to emotional eating. The military term *cascading system failure* refers to a failure in one area causing a failure in a different area that would not ordinarily fail. That is precisely what often happens to our eating behavior when we fail to maintain our exercise regimen and what often happens to our exercise regimen when we are not vigilant about our eating.

George, age 53

When I exercise, I am more careful about eating.

Justin, age 35

Exercise drives my healthy eating; when I fall off my exercise regimen, I start eating pizza, burgers and deli sandwiches. The combination of exercise and healthy eating creates great rhythm.

Exercise is not a part of the lifestyle of many of us, although we are hard-wired for physical activity. Not only is it good for us on multiple different levels, but after completion of vigorous exercise, we often will have achieved a much improved state, both physically and mentally, feeling well, balanced, and engaged. The resultant exercise "high"—a heightened sense of well being, alertness, exhilaration and soothing afterglow—can become so seductive and addictive that we can get to the point where we will actually *crave* exercise and where failure to exercise may lead to withdrawal symptoms! Better to crave exercise than junk food. And better to manage stress with exercise than eating!

I try to do integrative exercise every day. While at work at my office, I always try to take the stairs instead of the elevator (even up the seven floors), as much because I don't have the patience to wait for the elevator as to get some exercise! Instead of using the electric doors to enter the hospital, I use my arms to manually open the doors. When at an airport, I like to walk up the stairs instead of using the escalator, walk to the gates instead of using the "people conveyor," and pull my family's luggage instead of using a porter.

The key to integrating exercise into our daily routine is to always incorporate movement into our activities—it has even been shown that being fidgety is a form of exercise that burns away the calories in the form of nervous energy. My wife often resents me for this one (particularly when its cold or raining), but I always park the car far away from the shops at the mall in order to readily find a parking space, and walk the distance, not circling around incessantly looking for that close-to-the-store perfect spot. I never valet park my car if self-parking is available as it is a convenience that I personally detest—I view it as an insult to my health and wellness! When I am too ill to park my car myself and walk a couple of blocks, then I will valet! I must credit my wife with her ability to power vacuum, in which she works up a good sweat and gets good aerobic as well as strength training benefits. She also tells me that by mixing batter for a cake (an organic, "healthy" one) by hand as opposed to using an electric mixer, she can build nice "cuts" in the upper arms—in fact, people ask her if she weight trains in the gym and her answer is "no, I work out in the kitchen"! When I play golf, if possible, I will walk the course instead of using a cart so as to get some exercise.

Put it in writing and review it at moments of weakness. The legal premise of having contracts in writing as opposed to a verbal agreement is a sound one. Most of us, after a binge driven by emotional reasons, or for that matter—any reason—feel guilt and remorse and swear to ourselves that we will not behave in this manner again. That resolution, unfortunately, is usually a short-lived one. By giving our eating behavior some genuine thought, articulating our conclusions and resolution and writing it out clearly and legibly on paper, we have essentially created a written contract with ourselves. It is much more powerful of a tool than the verbal contract we have made with ourselves, and at times of weakness, it is convenient in terms of re-reading to help ourselves not lapse into a repetitive pattern of inappropriate eating. A website—*www.stickK.com*—will furnish you with a binding contract to help you achieve a specific goal.

To promote *disciplined eating*, it is a very good idea to create a written list of eating *diversions* and *downers*. Diversions are alternative activities to eating that provide us with a similar chemical release of endorphins and dopamine such as exercise, sex, great music, etc. Downers are the consequences from chronic overeating, including lethargy, bloating, guilt, joint pain, diabetes, heart disease, premature death, etc.

STOP before it gets out-of-control. The enemy of good is perfect. If we blow our healthy eating regimen and our best eating behavior, it is not the end of the world. It's okay to lose a battle as long as we win the war! We are humans, subject to all the imperfections, weaknesses and foibles that are characteristic of our species. If we fall off the wagon, we can get back on without losing much ground. When we think with a long-term perspective, we understand that a little deviation or detour off the pathway need not affect the outcome of our journey. To quote comedian Jeff Garlin: "*Slip ups are speed bumps on the road to recovery.*" We need to be aware and attentive, focused and mindful, and if we break our diet or regimen, not to despair but simply halt, stop and desist before matters get out of hand.

Justin, age 35

The fall is not a "fall" so much as a "jump." Have a few drinks, pancakes, or a nice dinner out—a rare over-indulgence is okay.

Jessica, age 26

I rarely eat when I am not hungry, but may do so socially because I am alive and want to enjoy the moment. I was raised without fast foods and an "everything in moderation" attitude. I tend to splurge sometimes on weekends by having a drink of alcohol and going out for dinner, but during the week, I am very disciplined.

Unfortunately, it would seem that many of us have an "all-or-none" perspective with respect to eating—an "I can't just have a few" attitude. We need to actively work and strive to break this often—fallacious thought pattern. We can cultivate mindfulness, restraint and moderation—our best chances for long-term weight management depend on recognition that it is not "all-or-none" and that we can indeed have "just a few"! Sooner or later, no matter how much avoidance and access control we practice, we will confront opportunity and, in order to survive and thrive, our best armor is the mindfulness to understand that we can live with ourselves consuming a moderate but controlled indulgence. No need to allow a spark to turn into a conflagration—and this seems to be where so many of us fall and fail. That being stated, the exception to this rule is those of us who are true food addicts, who must have a "none" relationship with our trigger foods in order to avoid an out-of-control downward spiral.

Andrew, age 24

I eat when I am depressed or bored. I have two extremes without middle ground—either I behave perfectly and exercise daily and the weight comes off readily, or I misbehave, eat everything in my refrigerator, stop exercising and gain weight. It has been a vicious cycle for years. I am often on good behavior during the week, but break my good behavior over the weekend. I then feel guilty and compensate by eating less and exercising more.

If we cannot do it for ourselves, then do it for our children. Our kids eat based on what food is made available to them and by virtue of the guidance and examples that we set for them as their primary role models. We do not want to enable our children to be overweight or obese and we have the capacity to empower the next generation with healthy eating and lifestyle habits. Along the lines of second-hand smoking, *second-hand eating* is a term that has been applied to the eating problems engendered in children of overweight or obese parents. There is no more influential means of inculcating healthy eating habits in our children than by teaching by example. We all stand to benefit. Additionally, by eating smarter and better, we will likely be around longer on this planet to enjoy our children and grandchildren.

Patty, age 44

The stress from my kids caused me to eat junk. I would binge—cookies, cakes, chocolate, from 6-8PM—to the point of almost needing to vomit. I was left with no relief, only a bellyache. Sometimes, I would eat for no apparent reason, seemingly a habit. When bored, I would find my hands in the cookie cabinet. My diet used to be fat, grease and cholesterol. I got to the point that I thought I was committing slow suicide and wondered, "who will be around to help out with my kids' kids?" I lost 30 lbs and now eat veggies and sugar-free, fat-free chocolate snacks. At work for a snack I might have a teeny piece of something, just for taste.

Close the shop. I like to brush my teeth after meals. Not only is this dentist-approved and great for our teeth and gums, but also, we are truly less likely to snack when our teeth are sparkling clean. Human nature being what it is, many of us tend to be "lazy." The thought process is: why eat something that would ruin the effect of brushing our teeth and then require us to brush once again—that would take effort and it is just as easy not to eat.

Maintain tenacity and patience. Our goal is healthy eating and a healthy relationship with food, which should result in long-term, gradual, modest and realistic weight loss, and ultimately weight maintenance. Weight gain is easy and weight loss is difficult, but the real challenge is keeping the weight off. Yo-yo dieting is an all too common phenomenon because weight maintenance is simply a more daunting task than weight loss. The good news is that anybody reading this is imbued with a well-engineered central nervous system capable of high-level cognitive function that can certainly allow us to control our actions and to comprehend that success is predicated on a modified long-term relationship with food.

Miscellaneous tricks—temptation tamponades. Putting a "fat" photograph of ourselves on the refrigerator will make us think twice about opening the refrigerator for unnecessary foraging and, if we do open the door, it may just influence us to grab an apple instead of a piece of pepperoni pizza. Similarly, posting a photo of someone—perhaps an actor or athlete—with the "ideal" body that we desire, may be able to influence us in a positive way. Another idea is to put our scale in the kitchen instead of the bathroom. When we weigh ourselves in the kitchen, we get some very objective feedback that can greatly impact our decision about what, if anything, we decide to put into our mouths. Just seeing the scale sitting there by the refrigerator is enough to ruin a potential binge! It simply makes the consequences so much more real.

Another idea is to create a thought pattern that will help deter us from unnecessary eating, as demonstrated in the following examples:

Rachel, age 48

At school, we have a faculty room full of tempting food for the taking. I try to avoid the room, but the faculty bathroom is immediately adjacent to the faculty room, so out of necessity, I have to pass through the faculty room a few times a day. So my thought is: the bathroom is too close to the food, which might result in the food being contaminated, so I don't eat it!

Isabelle, age 10

I like candy, but get mad at myself thinking that I will get fat or get cavities.

Michael age 61

One of the main motivations for my losing weight was the terrible pain I was having in my knees. I read somewhere that every pound you lose takes seven pounds of pressure off your knees. After 30 lbs of weight loss, I can walk and exercise with so much greater ease.

Justin, age 35

Before I reach for that tempting food that I don't really need, I think, "Do I really want to negate all the good I did for myself earlier today when I exercised?"

Remember when earlier in this chapter I related the story about the technique of "vaccinate and inoculate" regarding the tempting rugelach in the surgical center? An alternative "temptation tamponade" is the following: On another occasion, I was in the center, between cases, with a little free time on my hands. I sat in the lounge to read the newspaper. At arm's length sat a package of raspberry rugelach and another package of chocolate rugelach. They looked and smelled so enticing—how nicely they would accompany a cup of coffee. I read their list of ingredients that included palm oil and partially hydrogenated soybean oil (shortening). I know that these ingredients bear a great resemblance to the very atherosclerotic plaques that clog our blood vessels. I mentally pictured the palm oil and shortening obstructing my arteries and walked away. This time, mindfulness trumped temptation and opportunity.

Concluding Words

I restate my own goal for myself as well as for the reader—the integration of a mindful philosophy as directed towards the act of eating. If you can embrace this as your own creed or mantra, even if you use it as a general template and modify it in accordance with your individual needs, I feel confident that you, too, will be able to find your way on the lifetime journey towards eating in a more mindful, conscious, conscientious and healthy fashion. This will result in the achievement of the ultimate goal—a harmonious relationship with food—a powerful weapon that you will carry with you forever more.

I will attempt to eat mindfully and conscientiously, with purpose, attention and focus, recognizing that the primary goal of eating is to fuel myself with quality foods that will promote my health and wellness and avoid preventable diseases. I recognize that eating can be a highly rewarding and pleasurable activity, but as such, has the potential to be abused. I will make every effort to achieve a balance between the pleasure-seeking aspects of eating and the need for disciplined restraint. I will try to avoid eating when I am not hungry and when certain emotional states of mind give me the false sense of hunger. I recognize that this hunger, although perhaps soothed by eating under these circumstances, in reality represents an emotional need that should instead be addressed by an alternative and more appropriate behavior than eating. However, if I must succumb to the desire to eat for emotional reasons, I will make every effort to eat foods that will not cause me to feel guilt or regret, and will promote my good health and wellness.

Raw Facts and Truths

Most Americans are overfed yet undernourished on a calorie-rich, nutrient-poor Western diet. About one third of us are obese, one third of us are overweight, and only one third of us have a healthy weight.

The Western diet can be defined as the diet common to many industrialized, developed, first world nations. This dietary pattern, although highly variable, has at its core an abundance of red meat, dairy, refined grains, fats, and sugary-laden products. Processed foods, fast foods and junk foods are major constituents of the Western diet. High in calories but often lacking in quality nutrients, the Western diet has clearly been linked with obesity, insulin resistance, high blood pressure and elevated cholesterol, resulting in health issues including diabetes, cardiovascular disease, stroke, cancer and premature death.

Weight vs. Body Mass Index

An objective means of assessing our weight is by using a scale. It is important that body weight be analyzed in the context of height. One measure is the standard weight-height charts; these need to be designed differently for males and females, and with ranges designed for small, medium and large frames.

Better than weight-height charts is **B**ody **M**ass **I**ndex (BMI), a statistical measurement that compares our weight with height. This index is commonly used in classifying overweight and obesity status in adults—it is defined as weight (in kilograms) divided by the square

113

of height (in meters). The World Health Organization defines a *healthy weight* as a BMI in the 18-25 range, *overweight* as a BMI greater than 25, and *obesity* as a BMI greater than 30. We can calculate our BMI without a calculator, at *nhlbisupport.com/bmi* where we simply plug in our height (in feet) and weight (in pounds). BMI has been criticized for its being unable to differentiate between an obese individual and one who is very heavily muscled. For example, using BMI standards, many professional football players who are in excellent physical shape would be considered to be overweight or obese.

I weigh 155 pounds (70.3 kilograms) and am 5 feet 9 inches tall (1.75 meters). My BMI is therefore 70.3/ (1.75 x 1.75) = 22.9.

A subjective measure of our weight status is the good old mirror. We can scratch the scale, tape measure, calculator, and BMI calculation and think of an alternative acronym for BMI as **B**ody **M**irror **I**mage. So if we can be honest about the view projected by our unforgiving mirrors and admit that our body shape perhaps resembles that of the Pillsbury doughboy, then it just may be time to consider a change in eating strategy!

It is best to not let the weight scale rule our lives.

Yes, it is important to know our weight and Body Mass Index, but there is no point in obsessive overuse of the scale. The scale should be our friend and not our enemy. To quote Gil Reyes, tennis great Andre Agassi's fitness trainer: "The weight scale to most human beings can be like a Ouija board. It can start messing with your head." An idealized weight reading on the scale should not be our ultimate goal as much as an *active and healthy lifestyle* is. If this can be achieved, it is likely that weight loss will follow.

I tend to weigh myself about once a month. I have one of those scales that can give a rough estimate of body fat percentage as well. I'm not sure why I do this, but I jot down the date, weight and body fat percent. I suspect it comes down to how compelling and powerful the written word is. Most of the time, I can pretty much tell what my weight will be simply by looking at myself in the mirror, and I tend to fluctuate by only a few pounds, with a definite tendency towards a little weight gain in the winter and weight loss in the summer.

The apple does not fall far from the tree: Our genetics strongly influence our body shape and weight.

The blueprint that we inherited from our parents is of fundamental importance in determining many of our characteristics and attributes, including weight and body shape. So, to a great extent, our weight and shape is hard-wired and can supersede the influence of our environment. Although weight and shape can be modified through environmental factors including diet and exercise, when nature is pitted against nurture, nature often prevails. We can only do the best we can and we must accept that although nurture can be a powerful force, it is nature that ultimately holds the advantage. However, this is not to say that through strong will and focused mindfulness, nature cannot be overcome. I know of many who have surmounted their genetic adversities with a healthy lifestyle.

So, the propensity for being underweight, normal weight or overweight is inherited to a large degree. This is borne out by studies that have shown that obese people who lose weight will often regain the weight and underweight people who are forced to gain weight ultimately lose the weight. It seems that our metabolisms speed up or slow down to keep our weight within a narrow range. So, the obese person who loses weight ends up with a substantial reduction in metabolism and the underweight person who gains weight ends up with a gain in metabolism. These metabolic adjustments seem to return our body weights to those that are hard-wired in our genetic blueprint.

The formula for weight gain is when energy intake exceeds energy output.

Food, at its essence, is nothing other than *energy*. Life demands the cycle of energy in—energy out. A stable body weight is maintained by a balance between the intake of energy (calories) and the expenditure of energy. The laws of physics determine that if we consume the same amount of energy that we expend, our weight will remain the same. If we consume more than we expend, we will gain weight. If we consume less than we expend, we will lose weight. The simple but elegant formula for weight loss is for us to expend more energy than we take in: Eat less and burn more calories (most readily achieved with exercise).

As we age, our *metabolism*—the chemical processes by which our cells produce the energy and substances needed to sustain life—often slows, which can result in weight gain if we do not decrease our caloric intake or increase our caloric expenditure. So, in spite of a consistent and stable caloric intake and perhaps participating in some form of regular exercise, many of us will slowly and insidiously put on the pounds as the years progress. Some of the alteration in metabolism may involve loss of muscle mass with aging, which is one of the reasons why it is prudent to incorporate muscle-building resistance training into our fitness regimens.

Not all calories are created equal.

A recent article in the *Journal of the American Medical Association* by Christopher Gardner, et al., compared four popular diets: *Atkins* (very low carbohydrate, high protein, and fat); *Zone* (40% carbohydrate, 30% protein, 30% fat); *LEARN* (Lifestyle, Exercise, Attitudes, Relationships and Nutrition—55-60% carbohydrate, < 10% fat); and *Ornish* (< 10% fat). The Atkins diet, which has the lowest carbohydrate intake, was associated with the greatest weight loss and the most favorable metabolic effects one year into the study. Although I am not endorsing any particular diet, the take-home message is that the source of calories counts, insofar as carbohydrate calories have a tendency to make us fatter than protein and fat calories do. So, to our simple but elegant formula for weight loss, *burn more calories than you consume*, add the following caveat: *carbohydrates in moderation.*

As we age, we have an alteration in our body fat distribution.

Much to our distress, our body shape often changes as we get older. As we gain weight, we tend to put a disproportional amount on our midsections. Even the fortunate person who has had a stable weight his/her entire life will often notice that his/her body fat distribution has shifted with the aging process. The abdomen is often the problem spot in men and the abdomen, hips, thighs and undersurface of the upper arms in women.

Having a normal or low weight does not mean that we are physically fit, just as carrying a few extra pounds does not imply that we are unfit.

Physical fitness has everything to do with how much we exercise, and does not bear a direct correlation with our weight. (Of course, if we are obese, there is no way that we can be fit humans insofar as fitness demands a reasonable weight.) There are very lean individuals who never exercise and are clearly in a poor state of physical fitness; if they had to run a mile, they would end up incredibly winded. By the same token, there are very athletic and fit individuals who work out daily but are carrying excess pounds; nonetheless, they manage to achieve extreme levels of fitness, some even playing professional sports. So, to be physically fit involves maintaining a reasonable weight and achieving a balance between cardiovascular health (which endows one with endurance capabilities), strength (involving our core and other muscles), and flexibility.

Healthy dietary habits are a long-term proposition.

Weight gain is typically a slow and insidious process that gradually occurs over a prolonged interval. As well, weight loss should also be thought of in terms of a slow and gradual process. With applied mindfulness and diligence directed at a healthier relationship with food, weight can be lost in such a way that does not imply sacrifice, self-denial or hunger. Time races on rapidly and with a long-term perspective and the attitude that "long journeys start with small steps," it is entirely realistic to believe that we can ultimately achieve a healthy weight. The weight loss journey should be thought of not in terms of a sprint, nor as a marathon, but as a lifetime walk, done at a comfortable pace.

As important as exercise is, calorie restriction is the most efficient means of achieving weight loss: exercising restraint over eating trumps exercising our bodies in terms of weight loss.

This is not to denigrate exercise in any way, as getting moving and active is a fundamental part of any weight loss regimen. Exercise is incredibly important to our health, fitness and well being and can aid the process of weight loss. There are a host of compelling reasons to exercise, including the following: augmented caloric expenditure; aerobic and cardiovascular fitness; improved strength, physical conditioning and self-image; and a productive means of dealing with many of the emotions that drive eating. Ironically, though, burning calories via exercise will leave many of us with a vigorous appetite that can be potentially detrimental to a weight loss program.

As important as exercise is, it is not very efficient in terms of weight loss. It takes a great deal of effort to burn a lot of calories and the resultant increased hunger can often negate the effort. For example, I can run for 30 minutes at a good clip and burn 300 calories. By the same token, I could consume 300 calories in two minutes by eating a few cookies. When it comes down to degrees of ease, it is a lot easier to take calories in by eating than it is to expend calories by exercising. Therefore, as important as exercise is, with respect to weight loss, a reduction in caloric intake is of paramount importance and is more efficient than exercise.

Most weight loss programs are gimmicky, ridiculous, outrageous, unbalanced and unhealthy and should be avoided.

It is clichéd, but if it sounds too good to be true, it usually is. For a weight loss program to be both effective and long-term, it has to involve an intelligent approach that ultimately engenders a changed relationship with food. Gimmicky diets are unlikely to result in the necessary meaningful change in behavior that will enable durable weight loss. Only an eating pattern predicated on a healthy relationship with food will be able to provide all the nutrients needed while holding caloric intake in balance with caloric expenditure.

We have highly-developed brains capable of a rich array of feelings and emotions, and we literally bring our emotions to the kitchen table.

Our emotional status at any given time can certainly affect our food choices. The quelling of a negative emotional state by the *instant* gratification resulting from an unhealthy indulgence will often trump the *long-term* health consequences of such an indulgence. In other words, it is difficult to give thought to the distant *future* when the *present* demands immediate action.

The desire to eat can easily overwhelm personal willpower and public health campaign messages.

I have always been very puzzled by the "corpulence conundrum"—why very intelligent people who know better are either overweight or obese. Despite being knowledgeable and well educated regarding food and nutrition, for many of us, food can be such a potent seductive force that when confronted with the choice between long-term health and short-term reward and temptation, caution is thrown to the wind and we often end up caving in to our urges and compulsions. A mindful eating strategy can help us deal with this conflict and struggle that is central to the obesity epidemic.

Food addiction is not unlike many other addictions.

Food addiction shares many similarities with other substance abuses and addictions. However, unlike alcohol, drugs, tobacco, sex and gambling that we can live without, we cannot abstain from food, so on some level, we are all food addicts. No matter what the substance, addiction is a lifelong process and there will always be cravings that will need to be dealt with. To paraphrase author David Foster Wallace from his magnum opus *Infinite Jest: The sudden thoughts of the substance will rise unbidden like bubbles in a toddler's bath. The key is to just let the thoughts go—let them come as they will, but do not entertain them.*

Alcoholics Anonymous emphasizes that alcoholics are not to blame for the disease but must take responsibility for it—this holds true for other dependencies, including food. To achieve freedom from desire and compulsion, we need to be honest about the exact nature of the problem and arrive at the point where we admit that we feel powerless and hopeless, both from the addiction and the failed previous attempts to rectify it. We must acknowledge that the issue is contributing to life becoming, in some ways, unmanageable. We must do some soul searching and recognize the harm we are doing to ourselves and perhaps our loved ones in terms of our poor health. The process of recovery is about making progress and not about achieving perfection.

Eating demands solicitude and attention.

The ultimate purpose of eating is to provide us with the proper substrates, nutrients and fuel to sustain life. What we consciously decide to place in or not place in our mouths can make a world of difference in terms of our health status. Eating the right foods in the right amounts is a powerful combination that is capable of maintaining our health and healing. Eating the wrong foods or overeating is capable of promoting sickness and lack of healing.

Eating properly involves education, knowledge and a strong sense of mindfulness and attentiveness that needs to be applied to every aspect of eating. Many of us do not give eating the attention that it merits. There are many very harmful food substances that are probably as bad for us as tobacco, yet many of us do not give a second thought to consuming these. The Industrial Food Complex has created an abundance of processed food products that are seductive to many of us—sometimes to the point of being virtually addictive—which are heavily marketed and eaten ubiquitously, despite being unhealthy. Food should, on some level, be thought of as medicine, and the same critical scrutiny should be applied to the food that nourishes us as the medications that help heal us.

Weight loss takes a village.

We are all unique individuals and a weight loss method that works for one of us is not going to necessarily work for another. Some of us are extremely strong-willed and have the motivation, determination and perseverance to lose weight on our own. Many others will need to engage in a more formal weight loss program; my intent is not to endorse any one particular program more than another. Certainly, there are numerous, time-tested organizations that can help facilitate weight loss. We must consider the fact that if there existed any one absolutely fantastic, sure-fire, super method of weight loss, then there would not be so many different weight loss organizations, books and videos available. The truth of the matter is that in any competitive environment, "the cream always rises to the top"—what really works will become evident and will become a "game changer." In the world of weight loss, even though there are some very fine programs available, this just has not happened. And the real problem lies not so much in weight loss—which many are able to achieve—but in weight maintenance, a far more daunting and difficult task.

Having the positive reinforcement of family and friends is very helpful in getting on the pathway towards achieving a newfound, healthy relationship with food. Such support is equally important in helping to liberate us from the throngs of any substance dependence. As the Beatle's famously sang: *"I get by with a little help from my friends."* Additionally, one's community can offer many opportunities for collective support and at the heart of several formal weight loss programs are such social meetings. The world being the interconnected place that it now is, the local community is extended to the numerous blogging sites and online support groups dedicated to the effort of achieving and maintaining a healthy weight.

Warren, age 47

The competitive nature of Weight Watchers was helpful to me—weighing myself weekly and always wanting to weigh less at each weighing.

Advantages to being overweight (to be taken tongue-in-cheek!):

Obesity is clearly unhealthy; however there are a few "advantages" to being overweight:

- Less prominent crow's feet, wrinkles and nasal-labial folds
- More comfortable in the cold winter months because of more insulation
- More likely to survive hypothermia if your ship should sink in icy waters or your plane goes down on a snow-laden mountaintop
- Better buoyancy in the water
- Better survival when stranded on a desert island because of all that fat (stored energy) that will keep you alive long after the thin people have perished
- Less osteoporosis because of all that weight-bearing that mineralizes bones
- Strength because of all that weight-bearing—think NFL offensive linemen
- Built-in airbag for better survival of traumatic motor vehicle crashes

- Better comfort when sitting on tailbone or lying on vertebra because of padding
- More stable footing under conditions of gale-force winds
- Curvier, more voluptuous bodies
- More cuddly like a teddy bear!

Disadvantages to being overweight (to be taken literally):

- If you still do not know these, please reread this book!

100 Valuable Nuggets and Tidbits

1. Clichéd but true and relevant regarding the path to achieving our desired weight: long and arduous journeys start with small steps—it is not a race, sprint, jog or marathon, but a lifetime walk at a comfortable pace
2. Don't worry about a little fall or stumble off the journey—compensate with improved eating and exercise
3. Make an effort to eat only when physically hungry, not emotionally hungry
4. Exercise portion control
5. Food journals tell it like it is
6. Be calorie conscious, but not calorie obsessed
7. Goal of eating is satiety, not fullness
8. Try not to skip meals
9. Grazing is good
10. Minimize nocturnal noshing
11. Get plenty of sleep to help keep the pounds off
12. Keeping busy and productive is a great alternative to boredom eating
13. Eat nutritious snacks
14. Indulge with a small taste of temptation foods but try to avoid trigger foods
15. Keep healthy foods accessible, junk food poorly accessible
16. Read nutritional labels carefully—as if you were reading the back of a bottle of medicine before administering it to your child; be attentive to the size of a "serving" as delineated on nutritional labels

17. Try to eat the highest quality foods possible—better to spend it on food than on avoidable medical care
18. Try to eat as many whole grain products as possible: wheat, brown rice, quinoa, couscous, barley, buckwheat, oats, spelt, etc.
19. The closer to nature the better it is: fresh, unshelled peanuts trump processed peanuts, which trump peanut butter; oranges are superior to orange juice, which is superior to orange drink
20. Fiber is fabulous—soluble fiber slows down absorption rate of food and regulates glucose and cholesterol levels; insoluble fiber slows transit time and lessens risk for colon cancer as the fibrous materials "brush" their way through
21. Fruit is better than fruit juice, since fruit has less calories and more fiber (both soluble and insoluble) and phyto-nutrients (plant-based healthy components)
22. Unshelled nuts and seeds: unlike bottled/canned/packaged, they are unprocessed without added salt and oil and are difficult to over-consume because of labor-intensity of shelling; the act of shelling keeps us busy and occupied
23. Beware of energy-dense foods like dried fruit as it is much easier to overdo caloric consumption: raisins vs. grapes, etc.
24. Limit fast food and junk food
25. Limit processed and highly refined foods: beware of high fructose corn syrup, partially hydrogenated vegetable oils, enriched wheat flour, trans fats
26. Limit fats that are solid at room temperature
27. Limit tropical oils (coconut, palm kernel and palm)
28. Beware of consuming any chemicals in foods that are also products in moisturizers and cosmetics!
29. Sugar and salt in moderation
30. Avoid soda (liquid candy), with its empty calories and high fructose corn syrup
31. As a soda alternative, try flavored seltzers or squeeze a piece of citrus fruit into regular water or sparkling water
32. Avoid products that contain unfamiliar, unpronounceable, or numerous ingredients
33. Avoid food products that make health claims, since real foods do not have to make claims as their wholesomeness is self-evident

34. "Organic" does not imply healthy, low-calorie or low-fat
35. Avoid "mystery" meats
36. Avoid doughnuts and their ilk—the only healthy part of a doughnut is the hole (and I don't mean Dunkin Donuts "holes"—aka "munchkins")
37. Avoid preservatives in our food
38. Avoid hormones in our food
39. Avoid antibiotics in our food
40. Avoid pesticides in our food
41. Avoid bacteria in our food
42. Animal fats in moderation
43. Eat red meat in moderation, trying to eat the leanest cuts possible
44. Lean turkey meat as beef alternative for hamburgers, meatballs, chili, etc.
45. Try to substitute vegetable protein for some of animal protein in diet, particularly legumes—peas, soybeans and lentils
46. Try to eat wild vs. commercially farmed foods (salmon, poultry, pork, beef, etc.)
47. Good fats are healthy and filling—mono-unsaturated and poly-unsaturated—olive oil, canola oil, safflower oil, avocados, nuts, fish, and legumes
48. Consider olive oil as main source of fat
49. Soy: high in protein and healthy fat—edamame (fresh in the pod), soy nuts (roasted), tofu (bean curd), or soy milk
50. Skin poultry, because much of the fat adheres to the underside of the skin
51. Eat some fish, particularly those containing omega 3-essential fatty acids, such as salmon, herring, mackerel, anchovies and sardines
52. Use low-fat or non-fat dairy products
53. Use soy, rice or almond milk as dairy alternative
54. Baked, broiled, sautéed, steamed, poached or grilled are preferable to fried, breaded, gooey
55. Baked chips as opposed to fried
56. Drink plenty of water as thirst can be confused with hunger—jazz water up with ice, lemon or lime
57. Light beer instead of regular will save some calories
58. Alcohol-free beer and wine will save some calories

59. Cook healthy meals as opposed to dining out
60. Easy on creamy dressings and sauces
61. Order dressing on the side with salad, so it is not drowned in needless calories
62. Incorporate Mediterranean-style diet and other healthy ethnic foods—Japanese, Italian (careful, not too much pasta!), Greek, etc.—as Western diet alternatives
63. Shake it up by eating a wide variety of different foods as diversification will enhance proper nutrition and please the palate
64. Shop the periphery of the supermarket since this is where the fresh foods are located
65. Farmer's market as alternative to supermarket
66. Eat local—good for us and our environment
67. Eat mostly plants, especially leaves, as they are a great source of antioxidants, phyto-chemicals, fiber and omega 3-essential fatty acids.
68. Anything that grows on a tree or in the soil is generally healthy and nutritious
69. Anything that is naturally colorful is good
70. Artificial colors and dyes are best suited on palettes and canvasses, not in our bodies
71. Try to eat foods fertilized by organic fertilizers
72. Try to eat meals with your family or friends at a table in the kitchen or dining room, not in the car, while reading or while watching TV
73. Eat slowly, deliberately and mindfully
74. To slow yourself down, use a fork and knife to eat foods that you would normally pick up with your fingers—sandwiches, pizza, etc.
75. Very hot and very cold foods will slow you down
76. Use small plates and bowls to create illusion of having "more" on your plate
77. Use small utensils, such as lobster fork or child-sized spoon to help eat slowly and deliberately
78. Use chopsticks to really put on the eating brakes
79. Serve pasta prepared "seriously" al dente: I discovered this when my 10-year-old daughter made pasta that was way undercooked and thus was very hard and chewy—pleasurably so—each

bowtie requiring a great deal of chomping, slowing me down considerably and resulting in less consumption

80. Close the shop: brush your teeth after meals—this will help minimize mindless, between-meal snacking

81. Breath mints, chewing gum or sucking candy as substitute for eating

82. Eat as if you were dining with your cardiologist and dentist (or if you don't have a cardiologist, this is someone who you just might need if you eat indiscriminately)

83. Use a good quality bread knife to slice a bagel into four slices instead of two and eat just two

84. Bialy as a bagel alternative—absolutely delicious and so many less calories

85. Coffee is A-OK—tastes great, keeps us alert and focused, antioxidant; with a tiny bit of sugar, will curb our craving for sweets

86. Great snack: microwave popcorn, but not that processed junk—brown paper lunch bag with bottom sprayed with flash of oil mist and layered with corn kernels—fold bag and microwave for 4 minutes or so until popping ceases and throw on a dash of salt

87. Squash fries—great alternative to French fries and in my humble opinion are better. Take a peeled and deseeded butternut squash and cut with crinkle cutter, spray oil mist on baking sheet, sprinkle with kosher salt and bake for 40 minutes or so (Credit to Lisa Lillien, *Hungry Girl*)

88. Apple pie alternative: Cut apple into many slices (I like to use apple corer), put in Ziploc bag with a little cinnamon, shake and voilà—apple coated in cinnamon that tastes like apple pie (Credit to Lisa Lillien, *Hungry Girl*)

89. Carbonated cranberry cubes: instead of eating while watching TV, try cranberry juice diluted with seltzer, frozen in an ice cube tray; fill up glass with these cubes and enjoy (Credit to my patient)

90. Frozen banana: wrap peeled banana in plastic wrap and freeze—thaw and enjoy this frozen banana treat that tastes like banana ice cream and cannot be snarfed down because it is too hard and cold!

91. Greek yogurt is the best—tastes great and is really thick and creamy without watery whey, loaded with protein—*Chobani* is

my favorite brand—6 ozs, 140 calories, 14g protein, 22 g carbs, no fat, no preservatives

92. Sour cream sub: use plain Greek yogurt on baked potatoes instead of sour cream; also instead of mayonnaise in salad dressings and dips

93. Great snack: celery, baby carrots, cherry tomatoes, peppers, cauliflower, etc.—dipped in hummus

94. Great snack: fruit shakes—in blender: skim or soy milk, frozen fruit of your choice, yogurt (I usually use a banana as a "base" fruit and add additional fruit/s)

95. Great Australian crackers even though they contain refined wheat flour: Waterwheel Fine Wafer Crackers—super light, nongreasy, crunchy, delicious and 10 crackers have less than 70 calories

96. If you need calcium supplementation and want a delicious means of getting it, try *Citrical Creamy Bites* that come in chocolate fudge, lemon cream and caramel flavor—they are low in calories and taste better than candy! For a real treat, freeze them. I confess to looting my wife's chocolate fudge Citricals, even though I am not on calcium replacement!

97. Eat muffin tops if you want to get a "muffin top"—Dunkin Donuts coffee cake muffin: 580 calories, 19 grams fat, 78 grams carbs

98. Eat doughy foods if you want a doughy abdomen

99. Perishable foods with limited shelf lives are much healthier than non-perishable items that last indefinitely, as many processed items do

100. Happy ending—let the last thing you eat before sleep be healthy, natural and wholesome, like a nice piece of fruit—you'll feel good about yourself when you get into bed, and even better in the morning

Recommended Resources

Books

The End of Overeating by Dr. David Kessler
In Defense of Food: An Eater's Manifesto by Michael Pollan
Food Rules: An Eater's Manual by Michael Pollan
The Omnivore's Dilemma by Michael Pollan
Mindless Eating: Why We Eat More Than We Think by Brian
    Wansink
Eat This, Not That! by David Zinczenko and Matt Goulding
Lovin' the Skin You're In by Andrea Amador
Breaking the Food Seduction by Dr. Neal Barnard
The Get Healthy Go Vegan Cookbook by Dr. Neal Barnard
Reversing Diabetes by Dr. Julian Whitaker
Prescription for a Healthy Nation by Tom Farley, M.D. and Deborah
    A. Cohen, M.D.
Zen Golf by Joseph Parent

Movies

Super Size Me (2004)
Food Beware: The French Organic Revolution (2008)
Food, Inc. (2009)
Food Matters (2008)
Killer at Large: Why Obesity is America's Greatest Threat (2008)
King Corn (2007)

Websites

Diet Blog: www.diet-blog.com
Nutrition: nutrition.about.com

Physicians Committee for Responsible Medicine: www.pcrm.org
Center for Science in the Public Interest: www.cspinet.org
Hungry Girl: www.hungry-girl.com
Willpower: www.stickK.com
BMI: www.nhlbisupport.com/bmi
Food Journal: www.personal-nutrition-guide.com